CROHN'S
DISEASE

My truth behind it all

by
Leah Kobzan

CCB Publishing
British Columbia, Canada

Crohn's Disease: My Truth Behind It All

Copyright ©2017 by Leah Kobzan
ISBN-13   978-1-77143-308-2
First Edition

Library and Archives Canada Cataloguing in Publication
Kobzan, Leah, 1981-, author
Crohn's disease : my truth behind it all / by Leah Kobzan -- First edition.
Issued in print and electronic formats.
ISBN 978-1-77143-308-2 (pbk).--ISBN 978-1-77143-309-9 (pdf)
Additional cataloguing data available from Library and Archives Canada

Cover design by SelfPubBookCovers.com/Shardel

Publisher: CCB Publishing
             British Columbia, Canada
             www.ccbpublishing.com

*This book is dedicated to those who have
experienced living in physical or emotional pain.*

*May you one day discover
a pain free world and feel peace.*

Acknowledgements

I would like to thank the love of my life, Brendan, for his endless support and unwavering love. You make me a braver person and my life better just by simply being in it every day.

To my beautiful daughter, Blakely, for coming into my life. Thank you for your beautiful love each and every day and for teaching me what patience truly means.

I would like to thank my entire Medical team who has not only taught me a great deal about myself, but have also shown me incredible compassion, empathy and love. They have not only shared their wisdom but have also trusted me with their own personal experiences. I cannot thank them enough for helping make this book possible and ultimately being my prominent support throughout this journey of being diagnosed with Crohn's disease. Especially Dr. Coombs, Dr. Biggar, Dr. Oliveira, Dr. A., a Gastroenterologist Specialist, Isabelle Archambault, Anina Gunderson, P. & S. D., Massage and Acupuncture Therapists, and my General Practitioner. And those at my insurance company who deal with my case.

I would like to thank my family for helping shape me into the person I am today. For always being there for me and loving me unconditionally. To my parents whom I love more than words - you both have been indestructible pillars throughout my life.

To Amy and Trevor - I don't know how I can express enough my sincere gratitude for everything that you have given me and being there for me when I needed you.

I would like to thank my beautiful mother-in-law, Heather, for her generous love, encouragement and the wonderful support throughout my journey of healing and with the entire process of this book.

To my dearest friends who have been an inspiration, all of the very insightful people who have supported and encouraged me along this journey, thank you for helping make this book a reality.

Lastly, my heartfelt thanks to my publisher, Paul Rabinovitch and his team at CCB Publishing, for both the inspiration and unbelievable faith in my ability to deliver.

Contents

Introduction

I began writing this book because physically and mentally I have suffered with pain. I have become an expert in what living with pain feels like. I understand feeling alone and feeling like: can anyone out there empathize with what I am going through? It took a great deal of dedication to seek medical treatment and take on various health diagnoses that both physically and mentally were difficult to accept. This story is honest and it took courage wanting to share my truth, going emotionally deep into what living with Crohn's disease has been like and continues to be every day from my darkest days to those of living well.

You may feel as though no one understands your pain, and that reason alone was one of my biggest motivations in wanting to share my story. I hear many stories and empathize with so many people out there who are struggling. Struggling to manage their physical pain and masking their emotional demons. I have read many self-help and psychology books, but have never been able to really relate with how living with Crohn's is every day. I continually search to read stories from everyday people like you and me who are living with pain; I have yet to read any and this inspired me to share my journey of what living with inflammatory bowel disease (IBD) looks like from the point of view of an everyday regular person.

Are you someone who is living in pain or has just been newly diagnosed with an auto-immune disorder? Is there someone in your life who is suffering and you want to learn how you can be empathetic to what they are going through? Are you someone who wants to read a personal journey of someone living with an auto-immune disease disorder? Let me take you through my personal journey. Let me share with you how one can live well while living with what can be a crippling disease.

Testimonials

"This book is a must-read for anyone who wants to learn what it takes to live with an active Crohn's disease. It is the story of a woman who chose not to go through the regular medical road which would have involved surgery, but instead chose to be very disciplined with her food, her exercises and foremost who has learned to deal with her emotional being. Leah Kobzan's story is a great lesson of courage and determination on a daily basis. It shows us the extraordinary potential of the mind combined with an amazing day-to-day discipline."

- Isabelle Archambault, PHT, DO

* * * * *

"Leah Kobzan has small bowel Crohn's disease and unfortunately after many years of constant inflammation, she has developed scarring leaving a portion of her small bowel very narrow. This restricted segment acts like a funnel and does not allow anything except liquid to pass through it. She is prone to bowel obstructions if a small piece of undigested food such as a nut or vegetable gets stuck in that area. The scarring is now permanent and does not respond to medical therapies. To improve, she will need a surgery to remove that piece of small bowel. This will not be a cure, but for a period of time she will have few, if any, limitations. If we can prevent the inflammation from coming back after that, she could be symptom-free for life.

It is remarkable to me how limited her life and her diet are currently. Anything except liquids stick in the narrowed segment and causes her severe pain. As I have told her multiple times, most people would not be able to endure these limitations on their quality of life. Leah has taken complete ownership of her disease and has managed to adopt a lifestyle that allows her to cope. By minimizing solid foods and decreasing her stress levels as well as incorporating other alternative therapies into her treatment, she has managed to decrease her symptoms. The scar tissue, however, will not improve with these therapies. They are unfortunately a temporary measure.

Although we try to avoid surgery in Crohn's disease, this is the best option for her at this point. I do believe that her quality of life would be 100% better after a bowel resection.

I treat many patients with Crohn's disease. I have patients as young as 17 and some of my patients are in their late eighties. Everyone is slightly different. It is very difficult to generalize with this disease, therefore it is almost impossible for a patient who has just been diagnosed to navigate through the vast amounts of information on the internet to determine what does and does not apply to them. Having a good gastroenterologist who understands inflammatory bowel disease and who provides specific education as it pertains to the individual is key.

Although many patients, like Leah, want to take ownership of their disease and want to do everything in their power to treat themselves, this should be a joint effort. I would encourage everyone to do so with the help and guidance of their gastroenterologist. This is a complicated disease and we don't know everything, but as a physician it is my job to help Leah find a treatment that she is comfortable with and understands. My goal is to see her living a life that is not limited by her Crohn's. I know we will get there!"

- Liliana Oliveira, MD, FRCPC
Gastroenterologist, Inflammatory Bowel Diseases

* * * * *

"Fighting a chronic disease such as Crohn's, relying primarily upon natural means, is not for the faint-hearted. It requires a major shift in lifestyle, in priorities, in thinking, and in dietary patterns. But the journey is much like climbing a mountain: hard work, but in another way exhilarating as people begin to see improvements in their overall well-being. Leah Kobzan's book describes in detail one woman's journey along this path to health."

- Dr. Coombs, M.D.

* * * * *

"Leah Kobzan has been on her healing journey with a fierce dedication for as long as I have known her. She has had her challenges: mental, emotional and spiritual. A thoroughly human experience. I love how Leah shares her story to offer inspiration, hope and love in her usual generous way. Blessings and love to Leah on her path to healing and light."

- Anina Gunderson, C.B.T. and Yoga Guru

* * * * *

"It has been my pleasure to work with Leah Kobzan as her psychiatrist since 2009. From the start I could see the strength that would carry her forward... her intelligence, insight, and determination to face the challenges that Crohn's disease would present. I continue to be impressed with the hard work which Leah has put into understanding and modifying her chronic illness through stress reduction, nutrition, and exercises. She understands more than most why the gut is known as the second brain and how closely flare-ups in one affects the other. Through all the challenges she has faced she has become a new mother who is grateful for the present and happy to be alive."

- Dr. Biggar, M.D. FRCP (c)

* * * * *

"As the waves crashed onto the shore, seabirds screeched from above and the echo from my heart meant I couldn't even hear what the woman was saying. It didn't matter though. What did matter was that I knew why I was there and I was happy. 'Do you Brendan, take Leah to be your wife through sickness and health... I do.' Some people will never fully understand the depths of those words when they are said with purity and selfless love for another person. I made that mental choice long before I said them to her in ceremony making it official.

Fortunately most people in this world don't experience much of the sick part of the deal so I believe that most people don't truly understand what that means. Through sickness and health means that regardless of what any given day is like you will love, support, care for, empathise with, not judge and remain loyal and honest to that person. You will do all these things while dealing with whatever personal mental, emotional, and physical troubles you might also have going on in your own life. It means that to that person they can be present with you each day, be it good or bad, and know that you and everything about the two of you is real. If both are being honest, they can feel some comfort and peace to be who and how they want, without the worry of being judged or given an opinionated comment that wasn't asked for.

I love my wife. I love her for many reasons. I need not get into listing traits and all that jazz. She is incredible - period. She has been through more than I want to remember but do because I lived it with her. I did not experience her physical pain nor do I understand the mental challenges she deals with on a daily basis. I don't even slightly know what it is like to go through a process which heavily restricts our known and accustomed diets fearing for the worst and living strictly off of liquids for over a year. Think about that for a minute, but really think about what that would require mentally and physically to do. My wife has proven that she can be strong and strive to be a better overall being while living with a chronic disease. She has dug deeper than anyone I have ever known when life piled up on her and she picked herself back up when I feared the worst. She has broken down and rebuilt herself physically and emotionally while maintaining a zest for life only the super blessed seem to have.

I will not lie or sugar coat my life with my chosen life partner who is unfortunately ill. It has been and at times still is a heartbreaking experience, and stressful a large amount of time that is taxing on my mental state and body. This is because I have had to watch my wife, whom I live for and want more for than I do myself, go through agonizing painful nights and bedridden periods lasting weeks. I have had to watch her be so sick that I have wanted to take her to the hospital and felt faint myself from anxiety and worry trying to be solid. Solid like a rock. She called me that before. Her rock. I have had the best seats in the house when it comes to being out in public and hearing stupid comments or questions from complete strangers with regards to absolutely nothing that we are doing. Like, "Oh my god, that is the cutest baby bump I've ever seen," with Leah replying, "Sweetheart, I'm not pregnant I have a disease and I'm sick." I have heard and seen medical staff caring for her over the years treat her poorly or rudely for who knows why other than their own problems I guess, which she accepts as part of her journey. And I'm the rock?

I might say going to all the appointments and taking on the stresses and worries that come with the hospitals and tests alone is hard. Living day and night with someone who is suffering in pain and from a disease that is incurable wears heavily. I can remember times when she would be in the bathroom sick with the door closed and I would be outside listening to her cry and moan in the middle of the night and I would just lean against the wall and start to break. It's awful knowing someone you love so much is going through such a nasty thing and not be able to do anything other than be there. That has got to be one of the hardest parts, being there and understanding what that role is. Trust me when I say this. No one wants to hear what they should do or how to be from someone who doesn't understand what they are going through. We are human and there is only so much people can take. And I'm the rock?

I am teary just writing this blurb for her book recalling thoughts and memories. I know she is sick. She has been for a while and probably will be for our time together. She is my wife. Better said, she is my wife by choice. Therefore she is who she is regardless of what that brings. She is the rock.

One day she will look at herself, reflecting from something, and will have that moment where she believes it and sees it for herself and I hope I am there when it really happens. Don't get me wrong, I'm a solid guy but not to the extent of my wife when it comes to every day. Every day adds up quickly and it takes so much mental energy and a way of being to overcome the torture that must come with a constant battle. I really should thank her each day and I don't say nearly enough how I feel about her story and how she is truly an amazing person.

I have lived her experiences and know I would not have been able to get through some of the trying times I saw her overcome. People can relate to the odd tough time or injury or pain or illness but not to one that is chronic and every day. It doesn't stop, and it doesn't go away. For anyone going through more than they want to or not knowing what to do, know that there is at least one person who has pushed her way to loving all aspects of life. Learning to be in the present and live happily is so easier said than done.

My wife is a better friend than I have ever had and still I am learning how unique of a relationship we have together. Having a disease like this is horrible and I wish it on no one, but at the same time if one can learn to be and to love life for its simplicity like Leah it gives so much in return. This is something I am learning through her. I like the saying that says things happen for a reason. Leah has taken that saying into her soul and accepted her illness and is learning to live happily with it and its differences completely in the everyday world living with IBD. Being a part of her journey I know is a positive lesson for me, and waking up each day to see her face is the best and most positive thing that I can ask for to start my day."

- Brendan Kobzan (Leah's husband)

Chapter 1

What Is Pain?

Another sleepless night... I do not control the amount of pain or when my symptoms come about. It is almost impossible to know how long my symptoms will last or when I will be able to feel any relief. A typical 'flare-up' comes about when you least expect it and I have learned that I am lucky if it doesn't last all week long.

As I am sitting here typing and trying to forget about the mind-numbing pain that I am experiencing, I simply cannot. I worry that these painful contractions could be turning into Obstruction symptoms if they do not start to calm down soon. I find Obstruction symptoms are a little more agonizing compared to those of a flare-up. In these very painful times sometimes I feel as though the pain is never going to go away. In doing my best to exercise through the symptoms this morning, I knew I had over exerted myself. I try and push myself every day to get through some exercise because at any given time I can feel unwell and won't be able to do much of anything. Physically and emotionally I have learned that there is no healthier way to start my day off than getting in a little exercise, especially to help release good chemicals and promote positive hormones. It also encourages me to feel good about myself, believe in myself and ultimately remind myself that I am worth everything. I have also found exercise quite grounding and reminds me of what my job is. What follows is one of the biggest parts of this puzzle, my nutrition.

The worst thing I could have done this morning feeling how I felt, I ate solids for breakfast which should have absolutely been liquids. I was too hungry and could not control my craving. I'm sure it wasn't only because of what I ate this morning but the accumulation of things building. I love having my eggs and gluten free/dairy free toast in the mornings. That being said, however, the stinging throbbing feeling in my lower right side hasn't given me a moment without pain today. My abdomen is extended and you can actually watch it move. I have actually impressed my own therapists and doctors with this. Even now and on many occasions I often described this as a 'dead alien' feeling moving around inside of me. I don't think I will ever get used to this overwhelming nausea feeling either. On bad days like today, my abdomen is extended to that of a seven month pregnant lady. And trust me I have been asked when I was expecting. The excessive bloating ranges and depends on a few things such as:

➤ How much gas has been created and is still being carried in my intestines?

➤ How much active inflammation is present?

➤ How are my other health conditions affecting the symptoms of the Crohn's?

➤ What was I able to absorb nutritionally, literally that day or week?

2

➤ What physical or emotional distress are my intestines experiencing?

➤ What distress are my organs feeling and carrying with potential toxic overload?

➤ What accumulative stress if any have I taken on physically or emotionally?

For me and many with Crohn's who I have learned from, added stress makes a difference with our immune system and how it will respond or the length of time it may take to heal. Our digestive process becomes completely sluggish with added stress and takes longer to process naturally. Having a large section of my intestine already not working well, this added stress can really make an impact on my symptoms and the severity of them. Hormonally, the smallest detail can also affect me so it is imperative that I stay on top of my daily and weekly vitamin requirements.

My intestines feel as though a huge car tire is rubbing on and through every inch of them. I feel more sluggish, unmotivated and am having a difficult time concentrating. My cramps and contractions are becoming more intense since I ate breakfast, which does not feel good at all. I am also experiencing gas bubbles that can be extremely painful. Today, even though I do have a high threshold for pain, I would put myself at a solid 8.5 out of 10 if I was asked.

Growing up I dealt with a lot of IBS symptoms. However with this condition unfortunately gas is one of the most painful symptoms that I can face on a daily basis. At this point with my abdomen there are now loud gurgle and swishing sounds throughout my intestines. It feels like I have hard bowel pieces needing to be broken down or that are stuck within the walls of my intestines. I know I also have issues from having Candida which has quite a few symptoms of its own. I am experiencing mild to extremely severe contractions that have calmed down somewhat every 4 to 5 minutes... what a relief from every minute. Other than keeping my heating pad on my back, taking a hot bath or lying down with my knees raised, I just breathe through the pain and wait for my husband to come try and help relieve things until something subsides. These are really my only options when I am dealing with crippling pain. Luckily my husband is amazing with understanding the body, especially mine when I am having contractions. He massages specific muscle tissues and is able to manipulate my lower right side when I need his help. I am beyond grateful that he is not selfish. He is always willing to take the time and attempt to make me feel better.

My every thought, choice and action can define how painful or tolerable that day will be. It defines my treatment options and ultimately how motivating the day will be as well. I try not to take in too many outside environmental stressors which is not something I can completely control.

When I stopped working in 2008 as an Outlet Manager in a hotel and teaching part-time at a college, the grief of not knowing what my future held was very stressful. Being unable to predict when I would be able to return to work created a lot of anxiety and worry for me. I had no real focus on the day at hand. I not only felt different from everyone I knew, but to be on disability and labelled as 'off sick' felt like I was so different. I felt like no one understood me or what I was going through. No one understood how much pain I was dealing with. My husband was the only one I would trust to re-write my story. It is a consistent struggle every day worrying if my condition is getting worse or if I am maintaining everything well enough. It is a struggle to feel like I am consistently failing with my nutrition and food addictions. I also spend time worrying if I should be doing more for my health and perhaps paying for more therapeutic options. One anxiety alone comes from worrying if I will be going back to "work." Or worrying that my Disability Insurance doesn't trust that I am taking my disability into as much accountability as anyone could. A significant insecurity of mine was feeling like I wasn't good enough to get paid for having to take care of a condition that requires full-time care and maintenance.

On one side of things I had a long journey ahead of me, one that required I deal with a lot of physical and emotional pain. The positive side is that presently I have tremendous support in my disability insurance. It has taken time to really want to learn from different doctors, therapists and knowledgeable experienced people. It takes time to prove yourself so that others can gain your trust in what you are telling them. I also realized that I am not alone. There are many people suffering every day. It is difficult to hear about or even deal with at times. Most of the time I already feel as though I have enough going on, planned or scheduled. The assumption that I have all this free time on my hands was actually another huge inspiration in wanting to write this book.

Discipline in my opinion takes dedication, motivation and inspiration. It takes a solid everyday routine, accountability, energy and willpower. Discipline takes knowing and feeling that you are good enough. It takes feeling loved and ultimately a choice you make. Painful memories, harder times, shame, guilt, sadness, sickness, feeling not good enough, stress, lack of motivation, negative outside environmental stressors, stressful relationships or poor nutrition... just a few things that can keep you unmotivated, unwell or feeling unloved.

I feel as though I have learned what it means to sacrifice. There are many things that I have had to learn how to let go of or change for my own personal well-being. Whether it was school, sports, entertainment or volunteering. Whether it was intimacy, work or simply means of having fun, I have learned how to separate myself from certain situations in order to take better care of myself. I have learned to say no and protect myself from certain relationships. I have learned a great deal about respecting Personal and Professional boundaries. I have also learned how to set healthy boundaries so that I may flourish in my own personal space. I have had to re-learn and re-structure good behaviours with my nutrition.

Every day is different with how and when my symptoms can come about. To date it seems that I cannot surpass four to five weeks without building into a flare-up or getting into obstruction symptoms. At this stage where I am feeling right now, it is hard to describe how revolting the pain actually feels.

The hunger pains grow and my cravings are beginning to set in. Visualizing biting into something warm, crispy and filling... Yum! However I have learned that the worst thing I could possibly do at this point is to ingest solids or eat something that I know will trigger more symptoms. Any amount of processed sugar right now would easily create more inflammation and ultimately create more gas pain. Trying to have any simple or complex carbohydrates would increase the severity of my contractions and definitely put me on the couch with an even more extended abdomen. Weighing in can help guide me in knowing how much bowel is accumulating, and can make a huge difference in how I feel physically from feeling backed up in the Ileum area of the small bowel. It not only affects my digestive process if things are getting backed up, but can affect my energy as well because my body is already in work mode trying to get things processed. It can determine the severity of my symptoms and how long they will last because if my belly is getting more swollen this could cause a fever. Fine tuning this hourly balance of trying to manage my symptoms, accomplish everything that I am required to do in a day and stay healthy and motivated has been a work-in-progress since the fall of 2006.

Being sick more often than the everyday person and being labeled with a diagnosis has also provided an opportunity to grow immensely. While I continue to learn, mature and gain experience, I never thought about my life or took the time to analyze it in any real way. I never thought I would end up being diagnosed with an inflammatory bowel disease at 28 years old. I never saw myself as being physically or emotionally "weak." I never thought I wouldn't be able to handle the same workload or stress as others. I never thought that it would hurt so much to lose or walk away from relationships. I never thought I could be in so much pain and still have a fulfilling happy life. I never thought a lot of things, but I guess it has to work out that way sometimes.

What later led to a significant insecurity of mine as well was the feeling of having to justify myself to others. I didn't feel good enough so naturally I felt like I had to defend and explain why I was choosing to heal naturally. I would try to explain why I wasn't opting for emergency surgery or wanting to take prescription drugs. It always felt as though I could never satisfy a conversation with anyone. Of course this could have just been me feeling insecure, however I felt like unless I was going 'back to work' or going through the daily 'norms' like everyone else nothing I was doing felt good enough to talk about. Being newly diagnosed I didn't feel like I was able to relate anymore and slowly lost feelings for wanting to share the details of my daily life.

I am someone who has learned how to become very disciplined, and not just when someone else is around. I had to learn how to build a team of doctors and therapists to help work with me. I had to learn how to work with them to help keep me physically and emotionally accountable. This was a choice I made. That being said, learning how to live with a condition that is extremely complex is a lot of hard work and continues to be a work-in-progress every single day.

Although it has only been a couple of years since being diagnosed with Crohn's, I acknowledge and accept that there is no definite answer. I understand that when you're dealing with pain at the drop of a hat it is unrealistic to build certain expectations. It is not up to anyone else to carry my weight. I choose how I am going to live in this physical space, not anyone else. I choose to believe that what I am doing is exactly what I am meant to be doing. I accept and believe that I am exactly where I am meant to be, experiencing exactly what I am meant to be experiencing. I am a loving being and I am good enough to be taken care of as a beloved child of this universe. I am worth this journey. It has taken a few years to really accept what that means and was another beautiful inspiration in wanting to share my story.

Crohn's Disease: My Truth Behind It All

Chapter 2

Being Diagnosed

"Leah, as I suspected you have Crohn's disease." It was the late fall of 2006 and I can still remember it like it was yesterday. "The procedure went well and the good news is you have no polyps at this time in your large colon. We will discuss more in detail at my office with the follow-up appointment. Rest, take it easy and have a good day." There I was sitting in a cold unfriendly feeling recovery wing.

Probably makes sense for those who have had the pleasure of having a Colonoscopy and Endoscopy procedure. This was the voice of my very first Gastroenterologist Specialist whom I had only met once before this very painful procedure. Still feeling high from being sedated with fentanyl and Diazemuls, and while waiting for who knows how long to be told bluntly and without any real slim look of empathy, I'd just been diagnosed with a serious complex inflammatory bowel disease. I felt so sick and alone from the medications and the prep the night prior. I will say now, having experienced this twice, that I would never be able to do again the recommended prep method and will have to find an alternate way. I might as well go through an episode of food poisoning because the prep work felt the same in my system. During the colonoscopy the pain from the air that was being pumped into me was something that I cannot describe. It was very painful and I actually remember a lot from my first colonoscopy procedure. I didn't remember having the endoscopy procedure which I find odd. However my throat felt sore to swallow after the fact. I would have rather been less sedated to see what was going down my throat, but in the end I do realize that I definitely needed the pain medications more. I remember watching and seeing my colon on the screen. I even remember the second injection that I had to ask for because the pain was so bad. I also remember trying to cry out, "Please stop, ouch, stop…" I was really sedated, but could feel every bit of the cramping pain when he was close to my Ileum. What felt like a while later I could finally feel him removing the scope from inside, and then within minutes he was finished. I can still feel that colon instrument coming out from inside of me and feeling such relief at that moment because I was not able to go on any further. Moving from that small room where I was first having the procedure to the actual recovery room, I do not remember either. Still coming to and feeling somewhat out of it, I was really groggy and nauseous. I was still trying to wrap my head around what I had just been through and briefly told about having active inflammation. Waiting patiently for my time in recovery to be over, it felt like every time I would move a little I was going to shit myself right there in the hospital bed. I was very gassy and they encourage you to pass it. I was finally able to get changed, had a little juice, and then got out of there. After meeting my husband in a bit of a teary state, I was beyond grateful to have him there waiting for me. He wrapped his arms around me, and in that moment I knew it was all over. Within no time at all we were finally able to leave the hospital.

For most people the idea of eating after something like that is quite appetizing – also because you are starving from not being able to eat during your prep. Back then any reason was good enough for me to eat. I also loved going out and being served. My husband offered to treat us to lunch anywhere I wanted to go. I am sure anyone would feel that a huge reward is needed and deserved. It's mind-numbing to accept how much I used food as 'rewarding.' Now going back to 2006, it is with shame that I reveal to you that the first meal I chose to eat after going through the whole ordeal was... yup you guessed it... McDonald's! We took our meals, sat by the water, and with our salivating mouths started into our burgers and fries. I don't even think I swallowed two whole mouthfuls before I was sick. I felt it happen and I had literally just "shat" myself. How honest can one be? I looked at my husband and said, "We have to go home right now." I was mortified and all he really cared about was having something for me to sit on in the car. That way I wouldn't leave a shit stain on the seat behind me. Really!?! How perfect.

It was a few weeks later in December of that year when I finally had my follow-up appointment. Both my husband and I were very anxious. We were eager to learn more about what he had previously told me at the hospital. My specialist went on to say that yes, as he had suspected, I did in fact have Crohn's disease and that it is a very serious and complex auto-immune disorder. Specifically, an Inflammatory Bowel Disease (IBD). In trying to briefly describe how this disease works, he went on to say that not only does it affect the immune system but can affect organs as well as damage very large portions of our intestines which not only carry energy but ultimately absorbs our nutrition. The normal procedure was to remove the 'diseased bowel,' which in my case was almost twenty centimetres of bowel. This would help make my nutrition intake more tolerable and minimize the symptoms I consistently went through... so I have been told by doctors and some people who have personally experienced this. It was also briefly explained that this condition can also affect pregnancy, if we were going to have kids. The condition can also affect every part from your mouth to your anus. Patients who have an Inflammatory Bowel Disease are also at higher risk for certain cancers such as colon cancer and small bowel cancer.

The doctor was French, but as he tried to explain in English the best he could and knowing that other patients were right outside waiting... knowing that my time was limited and running out... all I could hear was, "Blah, blah, blah... Quoi!?" I was thinking this can't be true. I needed another opinion, and right away. Other than giving me brief information about nutritional information such as to stay away from nuts, popcorn and seedy things, he gave me a prescription for steroids and a recommendation for surgery. Our meeting wasn't too long, however we left understanding that Crohn's disease does not have one main cause or one main cure. It can have a genetic factor but nothing to prove that it is hereditary. It is a lifetime condition that is almost impossible to control, and even harder for those trying to maintain the illness and do it well. We left his office with a follow-up appointment for a couple months later. From there we made our way to our local pharmacy with the prescription and immediately started my first round of steroids. I was a sobbing mess. Thankfully, I am someone who has an incredible friend in life. My husband.

It seemed everything was going around in my mind and I felt completely overwhelmed. It was one thing to finally have a diagnosis. However being diagnosed was scary, real and hard to accept. Who wants to live with a diagnosis?!? Inside the questions went on and on. What am I going to do now? What is my husband really thinking about all this? Will I be able to deal with this? How am I going to get back to work? Do I need to talk with a surgeon? I was ashamed of feeling 'weak' and being 'different'. Also being labeled with an illness that no one really knew much about was also frustrating. I didn't want to give this condition any more energy than it already had. Probably one of the most difficult realizations I had to accept was that I couldn't do it alone and needed a lot of help.

I had just been promoted to an Outlet Manager at a hotel. The standards of working for a hotel, I cannot briefly describe, nor can I describe the amount of stress that I went through and dealt with every day. I was responsible for managing four outlets with approximately 45-55 staff. Typically I would work anywhere from 9 to 12 hours a day. I worked days, nights, back-to-back shifts, weekends, you name it. Some weeks I took no days off and worked through most holidays. In the four and a half years that I worked, I never actually took one sick day. My days off consisted with keeping track of the four outlets, and also the cares and worries of as many employees as I could, as well as the assistants I had to help me manage the outlets. When I wasn't proving myself professionally, I would be trying to be a good wife, partner and mom for our little dog. I would also try and be a good friend, a loving sister and aunt. Always trying to have the time and energy available for everyone.

Starting the steroids gave me almost instant relief. Within a few days I was happy to not feel anywhere near the pain that I had been feeling. I felt somewhat invisible and having any kind of energy felt great! Not having to worry about how I was going to feel after eating something was even better. I fell under the illusion that I was getting 'better.' Then what happened was I lost my worries in my work. I didn't want to think about my health or what I had just been diagnosed with. I wasn't ready to understand the overall picture of my health and how things were actually affecting my body. I wasn't ready to be accountable for all of my choices and go through the repercussions of my actions, especially those that would affect my health short- or long-term. I became somewhat of a workaholic and when I wasn't working I was thinking of work. It felt like I was living in one of those revolving doors, and trying to see clear in what direction I needed to put my energy, effort and attention seemed impossible.

Having to take steroids typically means you have

gotten to a place where you need medical assistance and pain relief. In my case I was doing a lot of damage to my body and the inside of my intestines were going through active inflammation. Having more active inflammation, some of it was out of my control and some of it – I have learned over the years – there are things that I can do to help manage the inflammation. There was also a good amount of scar tissue that had built up over the years, specifically in the small bowel area. Since this happened it is especially more difficult passing anything through that particular area of the intestine. In my personal opinion the side effects for most medications are similar. However steroids are a little different. I had to agree to take a steroid and was fortunate to have a mild kind prescribed to me. I had to take it for three months and pray that it would give me the relief my Ileum needed. I prayed that it would help bring down the flare-up symptoms I was experiencing, while allowing my body as a whole a little bit of breathing room to heal. The mental process around that was depressing. I realized that aspects of my health weren't good and I needed to do some work to improve it.

I was raised in a family where mother knows best and you only go to the doctor if nothing else works. I'm thankful that my parents stood up for our bodies and didn't subject us to many 'foreign antibodies' by immunizations or overusing antibiotics. We grew up on a farm and were raised to be strong healthy kids. I grew up milking goats for Pete's sake!

Working through the daily doses of steroids, I was flying through hours at work being an Outlet Manager at a hotel. I would work longer hours and take on more physical demands. I would have the energy to even go to the gym after work some days. I had a huge appetite and ate everything. It felt like I was somewhat 'invisible.' After a little while being on steroids I started to feel positive about being able to come off the steroids, which was within the next month or so. Even though I somehow lost much of my faith over the years, I was praying and hoping that things were all settled down. I prayed that I was healing well. I thought I was in a good place with managing the condition and working with it. I was going out for delicious meals with my husband, family and friends. Life seemed like it was going okay.

I finally reached my three month mark and was able to get off my first round of steroids. Going through that summer and fall of 2006, however, was difficult and physically draining. I tried beyond hard to physically keep up with the same momentum as I had been doing while being on steroids. Even though it was a three month period, I was able to get into a good routine with having added energy for that short period. While being on a suppressant the steroids masked most of my symptoms. By masking my symptoms it also helped to decrease the amount of pain I would be able to feel or have to go through on a daily basis.

By the New Year we were into 2007. I was on top of things at work and tried to continue keeping up with the expectations of my career. Coming off steroids I was feeling okay for a little while. However I got tired again both emotionally and physically, even though my pain would come and go or linger just enough to feel it through the day. I was not really being able to keep up with as much physical labour as I could while being on the steroids. I was masking every symptom with Advil 400's. As soon I would get any relief from the Advil it was like, what can I accomplish next?

At the hotel our chef at the time was teaching at one of the local colleges. I would go with him for a drive and check out the college when I could. I had been interested in this particular college and felt a real desire to be able to teach. I never realized that I would be good enough to teach others, especially at a college level. I didn't have a degree or a masters, nor was I planning on working on one at the time either. I then spent a lot of my time sending emails and going in to discuss options with the Chair of Hospitality. I was extremely fortunate to have been given his direct contact. Finally months later and in the customer service/bartending side of things, the Coordinator was looking for someone to teach in the first semester. This would be to teach customer service in the Bartending Program at the college. However I knew that I could prove myself that semester and then be eligible to teach in the Hospitality Program – ideally, the Customer Service Excellence course.

Needless to say, the beginning of the first quarter of 2008 was a very busy time. Not only was I Department Head at a nice corporate hotel for Food and Beverage, but I was starting to teach in an actual college classroom. I was so nervous and beyond excited at the same time. It was a bigger class than I had thought however – 55 students was a little intimidating, not going to lie.

Heading into that calendar year and getting into the flow of teaching, it was a little stressful that I would teach on one of my days off from the hotel, which was Monday afternoons. I really started to love teaching and being influential in other ways than just in my full-time job.

Most days I had energy for work, however having the two jobs was a 'full plate load.' I had energy for some activities with my husband, family and friends but not much. I didn't want to always say how tired I was or how much pain I was feeling because I didn't want to come off as being annoying. I still tried to hit the gym after work when I could. I had just started seeing an osteopath monthly for therapy. At work or not I am someone who spends a lot of my time on my feet. Anyone who has worked in the hospitality industry would understand the pressure and expectations involved, especially those who have been an Outlet Manager in a very demanding corporate hotel. I can't even begin to describe the emotional stress that I took in trying to be acknowledged. The pressure to be and act 'perfectly.'

Almost two months later the semester at the college was almost halfway over. I started taking two 400 Advil's twice daily just to help me get through my long days. I was responsible for so much and it was too hard to even think about giving up any control. I was not sleeping most nights and struggling to get through a regular work day. Gatorade, Frappuccino's and sugar became my best friends and kept me moving forward. My one off day came and went by so fast. Trying to be there for anyone or anything other than work was impossible. I was pretty rundown, stressed and usually very irritable. My husband was getting minimal snuggle time, which to him is one of the most important things in a relationship. At times he felt as those he had to even walk on eggshells around me when I would come home from work. However for me it was always about work, I just had to get to work and be that perfect shining example for everyone. Or else.

I was told by my gastroenterologist (GE) that it was not recommended to drink alcohol. However that didn't seem to stick with me once I finished the steroids. I wasn't a big drinker by any means but I was still dabbling in the odd bender. Letting go of the harder drugs I dabbled in just earlier that year, my cravings to party were still very much alive. That being said, I had also worked very hard to get into the hotel. I worked even harder for my promotion. I was hungry for the business world and my boss' title. I would take on any extra task that I could. I would help a guest or colleague out if they needed as well. I was there around the clock for my staff and proving to everyone that I was superwoman.

Before the college semester ended, a colleague/friend of mine suggested at the time that I could obtain this University Degree in Communications by simply using my business diploma as earned credits towards the professional degree. Of course, I was registered and had started taking courses within the next couple of weeks. This degree wasn't a Masters of Business or a PhD. However it was a degree nonetheless. Competition is fierce and I was a young businesswoman making my move and planning out my future.

That being said, at the same time while trying to flourish in my career and trying to teach college students, I was now also working towards completing a Degree in Communications. I was pretty much living in a 'numb' state of mind, masking the chronic pain and continuing onwards. Like so many other people I know.

After finishing with the semester at college, I was very happy to learn that I had done a great job and had proven myself to my direct superiors... as well as the students. I planned to move to the Hospitality Degree Program and teach Customer Service Excellence. My head spun with joy and it felt incredible.

Knowing that I only had a couple months off for break before I would be teaching again, I wasn't going to take my time off for granted.

That summer I went with my family and a friend to our family's favourite camping place, Sandbanks Provincial Park. I just felt different. Most of the symptoms were still very identifiable, but the lower right pain was mind-numbingly bad. I remember trying not to eat, but everything I seemed to eat just made it worse. I had the worse diarrhea and had to run to the outhouses every half hour or so. I can't even describe what that time looked like for me. While everyone was on the beach enjoying the day having their lovely summer vacation – I was living in what seemed like hell.

I only took time off in the summer because I lived to work and worked to live. In the early fall of 2008, everything changed. I got so sick that I was unable to get out of bed. I was in so much pain that I could barely make it to the bathroom. I went completely downhill.

I reached out to my colleagues at the college because being so sick, I was so worried about how I was going to be able to teach. The semester was starting in a matter of weeks and the prep was imperative. It was a nightmare. My colleagues at the college were so kind and told me to not even worry about returning for the beginning semester in September. They promised that I would be able to come back for the following semester and that my coordinator would personally take over the course for me.

My boss at the time was the greatest supervisor that I ever had the privilege of working with. He was a great mentor and a brilliant teacher. One day he called my husband behind my back. Humbly, he said, "Brendan, Leah's not doing well... I really feel she should take some time off work and rest." Later that week Brendan told me what my boss had said to him. It was then I realized how sick I was and that it was not getting any better. I couldn't get out of bed and if I did it was only to puke or make it to the bathroom. I smoked pot to help mask the pain. I could no longer mask what I was feeling with Advil's and soon after made a follow-up appointment with my GE.

I was able to get in and see him by September 9th, 2008. He advised me for the second time to have surgery. This was something I was not ready to really consider. I was petrified of having surgery. I knew it wasn't going to cure the illness. I worried about it spreading somewhere else in the bowel, coming back even worse somewhere else in the intestines, or having to start down the road of possible multiple surgeries. I also worried about the complications of the surgery. Nothing about having surgery at the time made sense to me. That being said. I know I was also riddled with my own worries and fears. I left my GE's office with another prescription for Entocort steroids.

Prior to meeting with my GE, my sister had referred me to a Naturopathic Doctor (ND) who specialized in functional medicine. Luckily, I had the opportunity to meet with him earlier that August. My sister Amy, I believe to be an angel in disguise. She stood beside me and was there for me in ways that I will never be able to repay her. She gave me strength and encouragement. She believed in me and supported me through many times, good and bad, throughout my life. Even now, I remember getting into her SUV after leaving Dr. C.'s appointment for the first time looking at the stool kit to have my stool tested for sensitivities... the hundred dollars worth of vitamins and instructions... all the information that I had just taken in about my health, and all I could do was cry. It was a lot to process and absorb. I had so much work to do with my nutrition. Having also now been made aware of what severe Candida symptoms look like, it was overwhelming to say the least. Trying a biomedical approach was definitely different, and I was going to do whatever it took to get to the bottom of what was going on. After waiting to start my second round of steroids and gaining further insight from this new doctor, he also suggested taking the steroids for a second time. He agreed that it would help calm things down immediately. In the meanwhile we had many tests to start, order and analyze. It was very clear that this was going to be more than a process. It was clear that it was going to be more than the ordinary way of doing anything I had ever known.

My new ND was a doctor who believed in natural treatments. He believed in the body and what it is able to do when you work with it instead of against it. He told me that this process needed a tremendous amount of patience, and that this process would need insight and love. He explained that this would not heal overnight, nor could we put any timeline on my healing. We were going to break me down and rebuild my health from the ground up. "It is going to be a journey," he said in a gentle and reassuring tone. And I was ready to fully embark.

I officially stopped working for the hotel in late August/early September of 2008 and went on short-term disability with my insurance company.

Chapter 3

Thoughts of Diagnosis and My Past

When I was first diagnosed I had family and close friends who were there for me. They tried to be patient with how everything was affecting me. They tried to support me while watching me go through so much pain. Looking back I give them credit because I was not easy do deal with at all. I would get extremely irritable if I wasn't on schedule with my routine, especially with my nutrition. I was trying my best to still fit in and be in control of the pain I was experiencing. I would try and hang out as long as I could and would sit patiently while salivating with hunger, watching others eat or drink whatever they felt like. I would forget about the pain because I would get so hungry from having to overcome certain triggers that if I didn't I would cave into my food addictions. While people were simply having their meals my mind was spinning with stressful 'what if's'. Even trying to make any overnight plans or to go away was impossible to even think about doing. I would worry about eating something and how that would affect me afterwards.

After being away from work for months I couldn't help feeling as though there were certain judgments associated with being 'off sick.' My co-workers were empathetic and continually reached out to me. However within a six month period I went from short-term disability to long-term disability. After that time I didn't hear from my co-workers too much anymore. I kept in contact with my direct boss and a couple staff members. The ladies from Human Resources were amazing and to this day we still keep in touch. Of course with my insecurities I felt as though they were thinking, "Who takes this much time to get better?" or "Why did Leah choose to heal differently?" I would think to myself what's so wrong with me that my doctors feel I am not able to work? The worries seemed endless. I was very hard on myself, so I assumed everyone was as well. I couldn't believe for the longest time that just trying to maintain my inflammation was becoming my full-time job. I had to work very hard to find creative ways to help get me through long days not doing my typical job and needing to still feel efficient. Learning and building any kind of consistent routine so that I could simply look forward to that afternoon or the next day took a long time. Yes, there are a lot of hours in a day, but when you're feeling unwell it is hard to stay motivated to want to try and do anything. Never knowing when I was going to be unwell was one of the main reasons why I was okay with remaining on full-time disability.

The severity of how one's diagnosis is measured or judged, in my opinion, is done without really understanding the overall picture. I understand that as a physician it must be difficult to try and treat someone when you don't have the personal experience yourself. When you have never gone through something devastating like being diagnosed with a medical illness chances are you will never really understand what it feels like to be in and out of hospital appointments or be labelled as being 'sick.' You will never understand what it is to feel like a 'lab rat.' There are many illnesses out there. However unless you have Crohn's or indulge in the same addictions and live with my immune system – unless you have my food sensitivities or have the same overgrowth of bacteria and deal with the same daily stressors – how can you possibly understand or empathize with what my daily life actually looks like? It is extremely difficult finding anyone, let alone an amazing friend, who can be selfless enough, courageous enough, and who never wants to miss a beat of your life. It takes an incredible being even wanting to understand what I need to do in order to have a few consistent days of feeling 'well.'

We will never know what someone else is really going through. What I do know is that I have been given a brilliant opportunity through every single step of this process. Life has ways of showing us many opportunities to learn and grow. I try to be honest with what I say and with what I do, especially where I am in my life today. Being honest not only to others but to yourself is a lot of hard work. It has taken a lot of therapy and practice, however being honest is a daily work-in-progress. I have lost a lot of my patience for anyone who is simply not honest with me. I completely understand how difficult it can be. Naturally, however, others' fears are not worth my energy or precious time. I just don't have the same room in my life for those who lie or say one thing in the moment but don't really mean it, are negative, judgemental, poor listeners or critical people. I have minimal patience for certain behaviours, and it's not easy always feeling like I have to protect myself... or when I feel like I have to put up boundaries from others' insecurities. It has been a lonely journey learning how to accept where others stand emotionally.

It can be very frustrating when people pass off having Crohn's as something they know because they get cramped or bloated after they eat... or read a little about the disease and then think they know so much more than they actually do. Crohn's disease, although I hate to promote its energy, hasn't gotten the awareness that it really needs and unfortunately doctors or surgeons do not have the only answer. For every medical definition that I have read – and trust me there are quite a few – not one description does the overall condition any justice. From where I am standing an author who has lived with Crohn's might be a little more insightful to anyone out there actually suffering from the disease. There is no cure for Crohn's. I have often been asked why I haven't had surgery yet or why I have not taken prescription drugs. Other than a couple family members and a close friend or two I feel the people I know well would be relieved if I were to have surgery or try medication. The assumption which I have heard over and over again from people is, "You'll be able to eat food!" or "You won't have to worry anymore!" Or if I have surgery they assume I will be cured, have minimal pain, and be able to get back to a regular 'job.'

Naturally people care about my well-being and of course want me to be healthy. Especially my family and those who are very close to me. I understand that it must be difficult to hear about my daily struggles and the pain that I go through. Ultimately I'm trying to learn how to become my very own best self and that is not always easy to relate with. I get that. Another huge assumption is that because I am often sick I couldn't possibly be getting better, so what the hell am I waiting for to go on drugs and have surgery? Yes, I have days of feeling well. Yes, I possibly even get to have a couple weeks where I am feeling good and have decent energy. Yes, I take advantage of fun activities when I can. Yes, I get to take in a little visit during the week when everyone else is 'working.' However at any time I can also experience a lot of pain and go through symptoms that many people will never even have to deal with. As much as I feel good one minute or plan for any social interaction, I can cancel at the drop of a hat. I do not have the luxury of having a 'day off' from having to live with an inflammatory bowel disease. I do not choose when pain is going to be present or when it is not. I cannot get out of bed every day and just say, "Um… what do I feel like doing today?" As one might assume, that is not who I am. I feel sorry for anyone who wishes they had my life living with Crohn's, especially because they assume it is merely filled with all of this glorious free time. I feel sad for anyone who judges me or my life because in reality the truth might be that they are just not simply happy themselves. I ask you, are we not worth tuning into our bodies? Are we not worth taking care of ourselves the way we deserve to be taken care of? Am I not worth the work? Is my health not worth every bit of my own care, love and compassion? Am I not worth being supported through my days while I live with a condition that requires full-time care? Am I not worth being paid in order to learn how to maintain an illness that I did not choose to have? Am I not worth the journey?

Another significant insecurity that I have had to work on has been to not care what other people think of me or the choices I make. I used to justify my actions only to feel good enough in other people's eyes. I wanted my family's and friends' approval. To be honest I wanted and needed everyone's approval.

I never saw myself living with daily pain that required a lot of specific maintenance, especially in order to not feel worse and to try and keep well. I am very grateful because I now live with such an awareness to my life. I feel as though it has been a blessing being able to heal, grow and most importantly be present. This has been a tremendous gift and one I would never take advantage of. What people need to understand and really get is this: it is not my fault nor did I ask to be diagnosed with this inflammatory bowel disease. I did not ask to be sick or live with an immune system that would attack itself. I did not ask to have a condition that is beyond complicated to live with or one that has no cure. I did not ask for Candida or to experience sexually transmitted diseases. I never asked to have such a hard time in school growing up or to be involved with inappropriate sexual conduct. I never asked to have my tonsils and adenoids removed or to have emergency surgery on an abscess/ulcer in my perineum. I never asked to spanked, slapped, pushed or sexually molested either. We don't always ask for things. That being said, this may be blunt however it's as honest as I can be. I am not caught up emotionally in projecting or encouraging my disease so that I can continue to live with active inflammation while remaining off work and on disability. I am not enabling my pain so that I continue to have all of this 'free time' on my hands. I am not a victim blaming anyone else for the choices I have made and continue to make. It has taken tremendous emotional growth to not justify myself and feel good enough about what I am doing every single day. It has taken a long time and a lot of therapy to just focus on the day at hand. I used to spend so much of my time not being planned or scattered, instead worrying and trying to be there for other people. Now I work just as hard in taking care of myself and no one is worth jeopardizing my own personal happiness.

Many people who I speak with wish they could have more discipline in their lives. They wish they had more time for themselves or their family and their friends. They wish they had the time to get more involved or get to the gym. I sometimes feel as though my friends and family are possibly a little resentful of the time that I have in order to help manage this condition and my life. I have come to realize that most people I know are so caught up in what others think of them and the daily drama of being 'busy.' In my opinion I am only a small projection of what they wish they really had or wanted. In actuality it has nothing to do with me personally at all. Even in some of my relationships people are suffering from not feeling good enough, wanting to be acknowledged or just trying to deal with their own personal demons. Most people I know live in this illusion of what they want to have, and judge or criticize others for their presently underachieved lives.

Growing up in my family we were always cheerleaders for one another. I feel that I am great at cheering on anyone and am genuinely happy for anyone's success. I love to encourage my friends and family to be their best self. I enjoy cheering them on in their daily accomplishments and letting them know how awesome they are. That being said, when you're dealing with tremendous stress and you're experiencing huge events in your life, your family and friends are the ones you usually go to for support. They are the ones who you turn to for help and compassion. My relationships have brought me everything from unconditional love, support and trust to living with added stress that affects my well-being. When I speak of outside environmental stressors, my relationships have definitely been one of them. People who are still dealing with their own insecurities or who haven't transitioned emotionally can be a little more stressful for me because of how emotionally accountable I have chosen to become. An example of this would be 'People Pleasers.' From my own personal experience they either agree with you in the moment but don't really voice a solid opinion on their own. They say things they think you want to hear in the moment however it's not how they actually feel. They come off as a scatter brain and do not ask or follow-up with any of the small details you leave them with. They love the attention that you give them yet they keep you at arm's length. Continually trying to put in effort, forgiveness and find the patience to hang onto to them, in my opinion, you can never build any kind of real expectation with them. The amount of energy and time it takes to try and have a reciprocal relationship is exhausting. Life stressors are hard sometimes and when relationships become clear they can add even more stress and emotional pain. Having relationships can unfortunately be some of the environmental stress that needs to be removed. Before I started therapy I never realized how much added stress I was taking on. I had enough to deal with and it seemed every aspect of my life needed change and improvement.

While working away on my career that I had been working so hard to get where I was in management, it took many conversations to wrap my head around what needed to change after being diagnosed. Why now? Why this condition? Why me? Did I bring this on myself? What did I need to learn? I just couldn't wrap my head around having to deal with a 'condition,' especially one that was so complex to understand even though it had now been a while of living with the realization of it.

When I was a teenager I remember going out with my friends to drink alcohol and have a good time. I would have to chug Pepto-Bismol to get a little relief from stomach pain when drinking alcohol. I would smoke pot or try other street drugs which always seemed to help numb my pain out a little. However the aftermath was horrible and I would feel even worse.

During college I mostly spent it in a 'party' or 'numb' state of mind. I had no real responsibilities other than school, nor did I have any close family around. I had left the life I grew up in and most of my friends as well. That part probably wasn't such a bad thing. Trying to just pass and get through college was enough to deal with. Forget about continually feeling sick and having abdomen pain.

Having to handle the pressures of living on my own for the very first time seemed hard as well. I also wanted desperately to fit in and feel accepted. I didn't know how to properly take care of myself. Being completely honest, the odd line of cocaine would help sedate the pain that I would often experience. I know... quite a ways from Pepto-Bismol and gripe water days. Moving forward and grateful to have graduated, I soon began my career at the Holiday Inn. Within a couple of years I met the love of my life, and then within months we had decided to move and live in Ottawa.

My husband and I of course chose Industry jobs. Being sick or not available to take a shift was simply unacceptable. From working right after college every day, stressors would build and we worked through it all. Eventually I would get so run down and really sick for days at a time. My abdomen would be so extended, and worse, really affect my lower back. I would have to just sit down at times and try to deal with the pain because it was so intense. I really have no idea how I worked through everything for as long as I did. Also always needing to be by a bathroom just in case...

Going from only seeing a walk-in doctor here and there or a gynecologist, I never had a family physician who I actually stayed in contact with. Having found a family doctor at the local grocery store during the next couple years after moving to Ottawa, I was very grateful for this because it was normal to come down with the flu, strep or bronchitis two to three times a year. I also had other medical conditions that required my focus because they had symptoms of their own. My stomach was usually extended and always going through some sort of contraction pain. I had been on the birth control pill from a young age so at least that helped with my painful periods. From this point it had been close to fifteen years of dealing with abdomen pain, different cramps, having diarrhea, going through bouts of nausea and feeling like my energy would come and go. Emotionally it was draining being sick all the time and going to various doctor appointments... waiting and wondering what they would say, unsure of what was going on with me and mostly living in fear. I tried to always work as much as I could because we were only working part-time hours after moving to Ottawa and could not afford not to work. The stress alone from our everyday lives was enough and even too much at times for me to handle. Trying to take care of the chronic abdomen pain that I was experiencing most of the time was very difficult, and of course for my husband too. I tried different prescriptions drugs, as well as Tylenol, Midol and took an Advil almost every day. I even tried taking this jelly-like clear liquid that a doctor had recommended before I was sent to a GE specialist which did relieve some symptoms. However they would always come back with a vengeance. I drank occasionally. I found that smoking pot or taking an Advil 400 gel were the best ways for me to medicate, giving me any kind of relief to help get me through the unexplainable painful days.

I got married in November of 2005. My health got progressively worse that year. My GP at the time had finally referred me to a Gastroenterologist Specialist, which from that point in time took another year to get in and see him.

I was grateful to have been referred to an experienced gastroenterologist. It was a relief to now be seen by a specialist who was going to be able to help me learn what was going on with my gut. Of course it wasn't easy to like him very much in those very painful moments when I was going through the colonoscopy procedure. However he was efficient in getting the procedure done well. One lesson that he did leave me with is that you should not have any expectations when it comes to your GE Specialist. If you get a great GE, you're very lucky. Now having been finally 'diagnosed' and trying to move forward, what later started to happen truly changed my life.

Chapter 4

Learning to Live on Short-Term Disability... The Stressors and Everyday Life

I remember the details of that fall very well and being back on steroids for the second time. Like clockwork, I slowly started to feel better. Before seeing my GE and making the final decisions to go back on steroids and remain on disability, Dr. C. and I discussed every option in detail and what would be the best thing for me. I will never forget those very painful days when I had been bed ridden for literally two months. I will never forget the loss of energy to do anything or being barely able to make it to the washroom, and going down in weight to 119 pounds. I will never forget how lonely I was and what It took for me to just get through my days. Looking back I am so grateful that I pulled through even when I had lost most of my hope. I was feeling beyond thankful for the steroids to start working and knowing that I now had a new doctor in my life who helped me to feel positive about embarking down what seemed like a very hard road. In addition to taking the steroids I was smoking pot, and thankfully too. It helped coat the achy feelings throughout my body. Smoking helped to reduce the intensity of the painful cramps and contractions that I would consistently experience. It would also help calm my anxiety when dealing with stress and kept me somewhat physically comfortable throughout the many symptoms I would go through. Smoking also helped me to sleep when I could not, which then helped increase my energy, which was very limited. I would have been severely anorexic if it hadn't been for the marijuana because when you're in pain, the last thing I wanted to do was eat. As well I became terrified of most foods and what the aftermath was going to feel like. The pot I was smoking was not legal and at times would just make me very stoned. We couldn't afford to be too picky either. Who can be when you have to buy drugs from someone you barley know in order to help minimize the pain you're feeling? Medicinal marijuana wasn't yet an option for me.

I remember when my family or a couple friends would want to stop by and I would get so frustrated because I was too weak to even talk. I didn't have the energy to ask them about their lives or give the details of mine. Having anyone call unannounced or having someone just stop by really stressed me out. Among other symptoms I was already dealing with, it was exhausting trying to feel 'normal.' I liked smoking pot and smoked pot most of my adult life. However at this point, I honestly wasn't smoking to try and get high. I was smoking to literally numb my pain and simply trying to cope with the everyday struggle of feeling unwell.

When I was working, the Advil gels helped get me through the day. However there is only so many Advil gels one can take. Being at home even in the worst pain, I felt that I could manage myself better than I could at work. Even if that meant having a hot bath every hour or lying on my heating pad. It was embarrassing having my staff always ask why I looked so sick. I had huge bags under my eyes from living with insomnia. I had lost a lot of weight and had to have all of my suits taken in. One of my servers used to call me 'stick chick.' I literally would go and stand by the oven just to get some heat at work because I would go through so many chills and achy pains.

Having recently started to work with an Osteopath, this was my first real therapy that I was starting to do on my own. At this point in my life I had only seen a hypnotherapist. I am fortunate to have a large family with loving siblings who want to help me or give me their opinion and advice. Unwarranted opinions and advice can be stressful but if I ask it is nice to receive. Two of my sisters at the time were taking Kundalini Yoga and were very dedicated to practicing it themselves. The lady who was teaching them was much more than a yoga instructor and social worker. I couldn't be more grateful to them both for keeping after me to go and check it out. Anina Gunderson became one of my greatest teachers. She has become one of dearest people to me and one of my biggest inspirations in life.

Having yoga in my life was one of the only things that I had to look forward to, other than my therapy work with my Osteopath. Back in those painful times I had a hard time finding anything enjoyable. Yoga was a different form of therapy all on its own. I would always leave the yoga sessions feeling so good about myself. I would feel as though I had just had a great work out that was much different than that of the typical gym workout. It was a time when I could focus solely on my spirituality. Yoga gave me a space to feel free and safe. It gave me a space to feel worthy and belonging with everything that was going on with my health. This was especially welcome since I didn't have too many options in my life that were positive or that I was able to commit to since I was feeling unwell most of the time.

Starting to show a little more positivity, I tried to regain myself and lift my broken spirits. I was feeling better physically from being on the steroids and having pain relief was good. At this point however, I was still waiting for all of my results to come back from the testing I had done with my ND. Starting a biomedical approach requires time for results and when you're wanting to feel better it could feel like forever waiting and trying so hard to remain patient.

As I was waiting to end my steroids, my nutrition at this point had not changed. Almost everything I would eat just killed my stomach. However being on steroids helped mask some of that pain. My body was starved for nutrients and my anemia was getting worse.

As we were approaching Christmas and before ending the 2008 school year, I had to connect with the Registrar's office to apologize for how long it was taking me to complete any of the homework. Luckily I was doing this degree online. However, it was still very demanding and stressful coming from where I was standing. Wanting to obtain this degree was a huge deal and at the time I wasn't ready to even think of putting it on hold. I would tell myself, "Come on, Leah, you can at least work on this degree. You're not working right now and have all of this time off. What, can't you handle it? You need it to secure your career." Looking back now I can see that I would talk down to myself, or worse, want to hurt myself physically by taking on too much stress just to feel 'good enough' and impress those whom I felt I needed to impress.

As I would make it through the long days it was time for me to come off my second round of steroids. I knew that these 'decent days' that I was experiencing might soon be coming to an end. This was of course my previous experience. Steroids are great when you're needing a very quick fix. That being said, short fixes or trying to mask the underlying issues – in my experience – simply do not work long-term. If anything, because you are masking your symptoms you are not able to feel exactly what you need to feel in order to be accountable for your health. There was so much going on inside my head. Finding ways to control my thoughts at times seemed impossible. I would get agitated or angry quickly. I had minimal patience even with myself. I was worried about my job at the hotel. I was worried about my position at the college and if they would actually even want me back. I was stressed worrying about doctors' appointments and what they were going to say. I was stressed out with not having any kind of social life. I was extremely stressed out trying to find anything to eat that would not hurt my stomach. I was worried about what people were really thinking of me. My family wanted answers, especially my parents. I remember my father trying to come over and help me one day unexpectedly. He just wanted to see me and help in any way he could. In frustration all I could do was tell him that he couldn't just come by, which led to him leaving and me feeling horrible. I couldn't communicate what I really needed from him in that moment. I wasn't myself, unfortunately only a very broken down version, and my emotions would get triggered very quickly. I also felt this way because he didn't understand that he couldn't just nurse me back to perfect health, which coming from a father, is all he wanted to do.

Being off steroids was a little scary at first, however with the work I was starting with Dr. C. I believed that his methods and approach would work. He had great experience and would explain things medically to me that no one else had ever done. I met with him early that January of 2009. As it turned out I had severe sensitivities to many different foods that I had been eating my whole life. The list was overwhelming to look at and took time to accept. Among the list of foods I was severely sensitive to, I was also dealing with Candida. We instantly wanted to remove gluten and dairy from my diet, and had to watch my sugar intake very carefully. It took me a while to understand that food was hurting my body. In addition, not only was I predisposed genetically – which played a role – there were environmental factors as well. I began to keep track of everything, day in and day out. I started all new vitamin supplements, even B12 injections, and everything from drinking Bentonite for my yeast infection to very strong probiotics that would help with the integrity of my gut. Trying to absorb nutrients was extremely difficult given my situation, and naturally it would affect me emotionally and physically. Like anyone if you don't feed your brain or your body, you're not going to feel well. In my case it was even harder because I was working with built up scar tissue in my small bowel and going through active inflammation.

I was very fortunate to have my sister Amy helping me. She was already working with her son who was diagnosed with Autism a couple years prior. Her delicious gluten-free, dairy-free recipes and cooking literally saved me. She taught me a lot and helped me to understand the medical information that I was receiving as well. She helped guide me in what foods I could eat and how to prepare them. She always made the best muffins and made sure I always had banana chocolate chip ones on hand. Yum! I will never forget how she was there for me at a time in my life when I really needed someone I could count on and trust. Amy was like a mother figure to me and I idolized her in every way growing up. I spent most of my days with her and her family because we were able to get into a good routine and loved being together. I was also very close to her husband Trevor who mentored me growing up. I will never forget what they did for me during the years.

As we were heading into spring, I was finally starting to accept the fact that I had to work towards completely changing my nutrition. This was extremely difficult to accept and even harder to actually do. I also had to take away as many outside environmental stressors as I could.

At the time, however, I didn't really understand what that actually meant.

Taking away gluten wasn't easy, especially if I didn't have my sister cooking or baking for me. I wasn't a cook by any means, but luckily I did marry a chef.

I slowly started to figure out a couple meals that seemed to work quite well with my stomach. Also my father had given me a book called *Eat Right for Your Type*, which had some great information. I wasn't at the point where I was interested in learning about nutrition, but I did some insightful reading here and there.

The days that I was living through were not the happiest. It was very difficult having to plan out every meal, having to wait between meals, and trying not to snack on all the yummy things I was used to eating. I became somewhat afraid of food because I never knew how I was going to be feeling afterwards. This was exhausting because I absolutely loved food. I craved everything and wanted to eat but couldn't. I began to mourn the loss of all the food that I was no longer allowed to eat. It was extremely depressing. I couldn't believe that for all my life most of the things that I was consuming were actually creating a huge 'war zone' inside my body and causing havoc in my small bowel. With that, of course, physically my body was always in a defensive mode.

My ND was teaching me so much, and brought a different perspective and relationship into my life – a relationship built on honesty and the choice to be healthier. Working with my ND was intimidating because he knew so much and had a lot of his own personal experience. I wanted to prove myself to him and that I could do as he asked. He saw strength in me and that made me want to strive towards perfection. He was more than just a doctor who would preach, he related with me as well, which made him very human and kind to talk with.

For the following few months I did my best to eat the meals that I found didn't cause too much pain. I was trying to get gluten out of my body and out of my cupboards. I was trying to minimize the dairy I was consuming, however that was very difficult and I would sneak this or sneak that. I was trying to control how much sugar I would consume because this fed inflammation and kills off good bacteria in my gut which compromises my flora. I wasn't able to eat salads or any kind of raw vegetable. I was even trying to switch to other nut butters and stay away from peanut butter which has a high toxicity level, helps promotes yeast and can increase food allergies. I loved fruit but wasn't able to eat too much of it. Eating anything more than a few bites would feel pretty uncomfortable. It was extraordinarily difficult, and I had a really hard time fighting my food addictions which had become very apparent to me.

Being alone all day every day and trying to find any kind of real discipline seemed impossible. I would do really well one day and completely fall off the wagon the next. When my husband was home and cooking whatever he wanted it was so hard not to want to eat everything he was eating. I would salivate watching him eat pizza, have a burger, or even a nice bowl of pasta.

My days were hard enough and after six months of being on disability trying so hard to work through very painful days, the expectation was for me to be well enough to be able to return to work. My staff wanted me to return quite badly. My co-workers also missed me because they had to help pick up the extra slack while I was away. My insurance company was waiting for me to return to work as soon as possible. At the time, I myself wanted to return to work and forget about everything that I had been dealing with. It had been a very long six months and I wanted to grab the reins and get back to being a boss. I missed my everyday life and the goals that I had worked so hard in trying to accomplish. I felt as though I was missing out on so much. I wanted to be part of a team again and be there for everyone. I literally missed working 10-hour days.

In reality, however, I was nowhere near ready to take on any additional stress. My direct boss and my co-workers in Human Resources were beyond gracious and humane. They recognized that my 'healing' would require more time. They never questioned my illness or the time that I was taking. They only ever encouraged me to get better and supported me through all the paper work with my insurance company dealing with my disability. Ultimately they also encouraged me to stop thinking or worrying about my job or any of the staff that I had been managing. I had proven myself in many ways at work and was recognized for everything I'd accomplished. To this day, I feel completely blessed to have been able to have had such amazing people in my life.

My short-term disability was coming to an end. I never thought in a million years that my doctor thought it was best for me to take additional time off. He felt that there was still so much work ahead of us and I was just starting this new biomedical approach. Results take time and when you are trying to remove many triggers while also learning to rebuild yourself, it takes time. Trying to get gluten out of your body alone can take from one to two years of consistent and very aggressive discipline. I was facing some big decisions and I was really scared. I didn't want to stay home anymore to take care of myself full-time. I felt that at least if I were to go back to work I wouldn't have to think about how I was feeling or how I had to be accountable with my health. I wanted to be like everyone else and go to work, prove myself, and become the next Food and Beverage Director… as well as a professor at the college that I had worked so hard getting into.

I didn't really know what to expect from this biomedical approach. I only had trust in my doctor, and when bad days came about I would question everything. We made the decision together going into the summer of 2009 that I would apply for long-term disability with my insurance company.

Chapter 5

Disability Insurance and the Headaches of Accepting Emotional Help

Through my own personal experience, being on short-term disability from the fall of 2008 required a good amount of detailed paperwork. The stress in having to deal with a case worker who would change from time to time was rough. I was extremely fortunate to have benefits. Having to get my GE to send in proper medical documentation seemed quite difficult and this would add unwarranted stress. My GE was very busy, naturally. My insurance company would be extremely demanding, wanting answers on a consistent basis. They wanted to know every single detail because ultimately they were paying me while I was off work, and from what I experienced from that point it was the insurance company wanting me to get back to work.

As I was getting more comfortable with Dr. C. I made the decision to stop seeing my GE for further treatment. With my GE I felt that I only had two options to choose from: surgery or prescribed medication. I decided that I would rather have Dr. C. be the one to correspond with my insurance team, as well as be the number one doctor treating me. He agreed.

After the summer I was set up with another case worker to deal with from my insurance company. This lady was very different from my first case worker. In fact I actually wrote her boss and asked if I could stay with her. Now that I was working solely with Dr. C., my insurance company accepted his documentation in place of my GE. I was very fortunate that they allowed this because my insurance company would give me a hard time when my GE wasn't getting back to them in time. This is not something any patient should have to deal with and it can add quite a significant amount of stress. The follow-up calls from the insurance company alone created stress in my life because I felt as though I wasn't good enough to take the time I needed to heal with a condition that had no single cause or cure. I was made to feel that because I wasn't diagnosed with an illness that would end my life, I should get back to work as soon as possible. What my insurance company failed to understand at this time was that I was indeed headed for a more serious diagnosis and needed all the support I could get. Going from case worker to case worker and having their own personal opinion added was also not easy to deal with. By no means were they specialists when it came to health issues or what it actually takes to live with a severe diagnosis. From what I experienced they are trained to obtain their business bottom line and can only have so much empathy for each individual. I was very fortunate to have Dr. C. filling out my documentation for them. The Medical Board understood better from having the very descriptive information that Dr. C. would provide to them. The minimal descriptions from my GE specialist were simply not good enough. My ND provided more than enough information and was thorough in his details. He began to follow-up with my insurance company in a much quicker timeframe. He gave them as much information as he could and I was very grateful to have him involved as well.

As I was gaining a little more experience about going to therapy, my sister wanted me to start seeing her new Osteopath who she highly recommended. She even paid and drove with me to my first appointment. I will never forget how she was there for me and how fortunate I am to have a sister like her. I was very grateful to have Sarah suggest this therapist to me because to this day I see Isabelle Archambault without fail every month. She is an incredible therapist and phenomenal person. She has been nothing but a gift and a true blessing in my life. She has become a very special friend. I admire her dearly and continue to look up to her as one of my teachers.

Having already been doing yoga on Friday mornings with Ms. Anina for the past little while, I also started to see her for short counselling sessions as well. I was willing to try as many different forms of therapy as I could.

As I mentioned, I come from a big family. My sister Amy had also referred me to her massage therapist. This women was so kind and I couldn't have had a more competent massage therapist. Seeing her for massage therapy gave me such a wonderful release from all of the accumulative tension in my body. She is a kindred spirit and absolutely one of the most beautiful people I have ever met. I added her to my team and started seeing her on a monthly basis for massage therapy. It felt really nice to have three women in my life who were encouraging, loving and only wanted the best for me. Having these therapists in my life allowed me to have an allocated time where the focus was solely on me, my health, and to be able to be in touch with how I was feeling physically and emotionally. It empowered me to be better and strive towards healing the root causes of this illness. I only felt support, trust and encouragement.

There was a lot that was starting to happen heading into the fall of 2009. My husband and I were looking for our first home to buy. It was strongly suggested to me by my doctors to avoid additional stress, but this was hard to avoid going through my everyday life, let alone the details and stress of buying a new home. We never thought we would have an opportunity to buy a home at that point in our lives. However because of very sad circumstances within my husband's family, we were able to purchase our first home in September 2009.

I remember the very first day we moved in, and naturally I wanted to celebrate. So what did I ask my sister to bring us? Something to eat? Yup, that's right, poutine and a can of coke. One of my absolute favourites. Every occasion seemed to be another reason for me to eat or cheat. There was always a reason to eat and take in a little fried starch, gluten or dairy. Or better yet sugar treats like chocolate bars or Blizzards from Dairy Queen, despite the fact that I was told such foods were severely hurting my body. Yes, it was on my mind when I would pick up the fork, however I did not have enough self-worth, self-control or self-discipline to have such restrictions with my nutrition. It was like getting on a rollercoaster that never ended. I always felt like I deserved a treat because of all the good work that I was doing. I felt like I deserved the food as a reward because of how much I had to deal with even simply living with the diagnosis of an illness. I was a victim in life, and emotionally food made me happy. I always craved food and worse were carbohydrates, dairy products and anything with sugar. There were also so many memories related to different cheat foods: Thanksgiving and having to have lemon meringue pie, or Halloween – who can't eat candy on Halloween? I had somehow gone from a somewhat healthy farm girl to someone living with severe food addictions. I was masking so many of my emotions, worries and fears by eating. If I had a really bad day, I would tell myself it was okay to eat the things that I really shouldn't have been eating just to feel better in that moment. I hated watching everyone else eat everything they wanted and not feeling chronic pain afterwards. It was beyond frustrating, and to feel better I would eat what I was craving. I justified it to myself somehow and would just deal with the pain as the result. That sadly felt normal for me. I wasn't paying attention to the overall picture. I was still only seeing a couple feet in front of me. I would dream about every kind of food. I would picture how it would taste. I would count down hours until I could eat again. After not being able to eat for days at a time when I was in pain, that would also really mess me up and made my cravings worse.

After seeing Dr. C. and spending a lot of time discussing how I was doing, I had to be honest with how much I was struggling with my nutrition. He was very aware because not only could he see my destructive self emotionally falling apart when we would be going through an appointment, but he also saw my results with how I was doing through different blood work, CT scans, ultrasounds and the MRI results.

It wasn't easy trying to explain how painful bouts would come about. I would have a good couple of days, but when anything would even 'trigger' me emotionally I would turn to food... and at times even drugs or alcohol. Clearly I had addictions that needed to be addressed. To this day I am still trying to figure out if I had learned this behaviour from a young age somehow... especially with food. It was also clear that I was suffering from some emotional trauma. Ultimately I needed more help with this because I was a ticking time bomb. I was filled with guilt, anger, resentment, low self-esteem and feelings of unworthiness. I was soon referred to a wonderful psychiatrist named Dr. B. She was recommended by Dr. C., and we talked about seeing her together and discussed why this might be helpful. I was starting to trust in the medical process, and I knew my inner worth needed saving if I was ever going to become strong enough to heal and make healthier choices for myself. My second brain – being the 'gut' – was getting good attention, however my emotions and mental health were not. I chose to let go of my judgments and insecurities with seeing a 'shrink.' I knew inside that it was only fear I felt about what the therapist was going to think of me or say on paper. This was a behaviour I wanted to change to become more courageous and live by my own integrity. I fully agreed with Dr. C. that this was simply another way I could seek additional help. I started full-time therapy with a psychiatrist named Dr. B. in the late fall of 2009.

In the spring of 2010 I was starting to get used to having a 'team' whom I would work with. Doctors and therapists who I was now working with on a consistent basis. I struggled through most of my days, however since it was almost two years later I began to take my diagnosis a little more seriously and I needed to as well. I hated being in so much pain, especially after I would eat. I also overate most of the time because I never knew when I would be able to eat again. Being honest, it made me happy so there was no real limit to how much I could eat at one time. It fulfilled me and felt good in the moment. I finally starting accepting that I could not eat any more gluten. I wasn't ready to accept the other major sensitivities that I needed to, but at least I was ready to start taking the gluten sensitivities seriously. I, of course, allowed myself fries from restaurants or from chip trucks that were cooked in the same oil as those products with gluten. It was a starting point however.

While still trying to study my Communications Degree through University, I needed more help than I realized. I would ask my sisters to help me with whatever they could on my papers or to proofread my work. One aspect of it was that I didn't have the energy or concentration, and was always sick dealing with all my symptoms. The other part was that I did not learn a solid work ethic around homework or had the discipline, and was never a really strong student academically. Gym came naturally for me, and if we could get through high school with our athletic abilities, that would have been the golden ticket for me. I had a couple years of high school where I actually graduated with decent grades... well I guess great grades for me. However most of my life I was a poor student. I almost failed grade 6 and probably would have failed grade 10 as well if it hadn't been for my mother. Looking back it was embarrassing for me. I would always prefer to ask others for their work even if I knew the answer or wanted to put my hand up. I just wasn't confident enough and always second guessed myself. My self-worth and self-esteem were very low and I never learned another way to be. I always needed the approval or opinion from someone else. Having the ability is one thing, but having a good work ethic, discipline, loving encouragement and academic support is another.

I carried on with my studies and continued to carry the weight of wanting to finish my professional degree in Communications.

Trying desperately to seek out any and all medical treatments I could use to help reduce the amount of pain I was living with, finally in the late fall of 2010 I was approved for medicinal marijuana. Health Canada was finally on board with supporting those who lived with chronic illnesses. I had to, of course, work out any and all of my emotional reasoning with my physiatrist. I had to keep myself accountable to a certain amount and discuss with my doctors during every visit. I went from smoking pot just to smoke and help take the edge off, to then smoking to numb myself and mask my symptoms, to finally smoking around my meal periods and when I felt it was appropriate. I was only willing to heal with natural medicine as much as I could. I didn't realize how many beneficial medicinal properties were found from medical weed. I was going through so many symptoms and didn't want to have to take everyday drugs to suppress my immune system. There aren't many other natural options made available for patients. Health Canada had very strict guidelines and they required a lot of medical information from my doctors. However my medical team felt this was a good solution to help me manage my very painful days. This allowed me to regain some energy back into my life. It also helped my concentration level and kept me in a less tense state of being, both physically and emotionally. I was never someone who could appreciate just being in the moment without many thoughts or worries circulating in my mind. Unless you have experienced smoking regular street grade weed to having the privilege of trying a medicinal grade weed, I can say that the difference is night and day. It would be beyond helpful if more doctors and therapists had to experience it for themselves so they could move away from the judgment associated with assuming it is anything like regular street grade drugs. Having a product that is grown in a clean and proper environment with organic nutrients, grown with care, flushed waste and salts, is very different than a product grown in a dirty, moldy, hidden area with poor fertilizers and chemicals added to help give a strong effect and do not produce the same grade or quality marijuana.

It is important to understand the medicinal properties

and how much they can benefit patients when one is looking and wanting more of a natural treatment with fewer side effects. Unfortunately, however, one feeling did continually come over me and that was shame. Feeling shamed because my treatment wasn't considered the 'norm' and I chose to smoke medicinal weed over taking suppressants. The difference in the long-term effects comparing the use of typical pharmaceutical drugs compared to medicinal marijuana is quite amazing if you took the time to actually look at it.

In my opinion, unless a person gains personal experience or insight with using medicinal grade marijuana or chooses to educate themselves fully to understand its potential benefits, they have no grounds to judge or criticize anyone who chooses to smoke medicinal weed for their own personal medical journey.

Chapter 6

The Process of Short-Term Disability

In early March 2011 I received documentation from my insurance company saying that they were requesting an Independent Medical Assessment. They set up two different appointments for me to attend, one with a GE specialist that was two hours away and the other with a Psychologist whose office was right in Ottawa. The letter stated that this was mandatory as part of being on disability with my insurance company. I understood their policy, however it is never easy having to share your life and health journey with a complete stranger. This is especially true when people you don't even know get to read the results before you do. Adding to that matter, in the last paragraph of the letter they added: "Your monthly payments will continue while we wait for the results of your assessment. Your case worker will call you after he reviews the report." I always carried this fear and worried that I would have to be strong enough at any time just in case I would no longer receive an income from my disability. This only added unwarranted stress. At the time this case worker was now the third case worker since being on disability. Let me just say he was very aggressive in how he managed my case. After I was unable to make the assessment for the GE far away from my home, he literally caused me to go through so much anxiety while on the phone with him that I had to call my therapist just to calm down. Trying to explain your broken health to someone who is not sick and has no actual experience or clue what it is like to be sick all the time, let me know tell you is very stressful. It is like they are being paid to prove you are lying your way through the system.

Early that April I received another letter from my insurance company. It stated: "This letter is to let you know that you are approaching a change in your plan definition of disability that may affect whether you will continue to receive benefits." Reading this paragraph alone raised my anxiety and right away I felt very stressed. Being on short-term disability since the fall of 2008, I felt like I had failed in some way because I wasn't well enough to go back to my full-time job. Even worse, I wasn't choosing to heal in the typical way that most people with Crohn's disease had chosen. I felt as though I always had to prove myself and the course of treatments, exams and procedures, even though I was already going through a lot and just trying to not be so sick all the time.

Living every day with different symptoms and various pains isn't a path most people would want to be on, especially when symptoms and pains can vary from moderate to severe and never knowing how long or intense they would be. I never imagined a life in which this would become my full-time job in which I would be trying to manage.

In the past I was someone who looked for the quickest treatment possible. Anything over the counter, street drugs, even alcohol could help numb out the pain at times. However living with a diagnosis I can say does change how I have had to really look at my health. Even though I can only try to explain some of the different symptoms that I face on a daily basis, here is what I can describe about them. They can range from having moderate to severe abdominal pain, gas build up, bloating, very sharp 'binding' like sensations throughout my intestines and especially in my right lower side. Abdominal cramping and contractions that can range from mild to extremely intense in minutes. Spasms that can sometimes be just paralyzing. I build up fevers that can start rapidly when my immune system has taken on too much strain, stress or certain food solids that get built up in a very narrowed, obstructed piece of my intestine. There is only a 'straw-like' space going through a section of my intestine for things to process through and can cause very painful symptoms, flare-ups and obstruction pain. In these cases these can last from days to a full week. I consistently have a distended belly that makes loud gas and gurgle sounds. I often experience lower back pain from having an extended belly, mostly after I eat. At times solids make my life very painful. I can often have bowel movements many times throughout the day and night. I can experience vaginal bleeding and some anal bleeding, which depends on what is going on inside my intestinal track or if I'm experiencing ulcers. I also had an ulcer and abscess surgery in my perineum area when I was younger. Dealing with it being activated on and off over the years I often experience a build-up of fluid or some leakage, which depending on my bowel state, can be extremely painful. I often experience nausea which can cause vomiting at times, and even more so if I have consumed too many solids and they are not passing through my restricted area. This segment of bowel is my 'diseased bowel.' I also live with chronic fatigue. Chronic fatigue is persistent fatigue, resulting from dealing with chronic pain, and sleep disturbances which is why insomnia can vary. Adding to those symptoms are neurologic autonomic and immune dysfunction. Why my insomnia varies is because I get woken up by uncontrollable pain and this obviously affects my sleep pattern. Having trouble sleeping on a consistent basis can also affect my concentration and mood for the next day or two. During menstruation there is additional pressure, contractions and cramps that I will often experience. Most times I will wear panty liners all day and night, worrying about some kind of uncontrollable bowel accident. This is in addition to also worrying about potential leakage from my surgery site in my perineum area. Another caution about living with IBD is that when needed I have to use a bathroom right away because not only can I lose control of the muscles, but this adds additional pressure causing additional pain if stool and gas are backed up.

Another health related condition and impairment that I have and go through are food intolerances that are known to have negative reactions and effects on my immune system. These 'unfriendly' foods entering my system can cause unpleasant feelings, some being extreme. I was unaware of this until my ND had my stool tested.

Here are some comments regarding just a couple of my main intolerances from a lab and their interpretation of fecal Anti-tissue Transglutaminase: "You have an auto-immune reaction to the human enzyme tissue transglutaminase, secondary to dietary gluten sensitivity. Interpretation of HLA-DQ Testing: Although you do not possess the main HLA-DQB1 genes predisposing to celiac sprue (HLA-DQB1*0201 or HLA-DQB1*0302), HLA gene analysis reveals that you have two copies of a gene that predisposes to gluten sensitivity (any DQ1, DQ2 not by HLA-DQB1*0201, or DQ3 not by HLA-DQB1*0302). Having two copies of a gluten sensitivity gene means that each of your parents and all of your children will possess at least one copy of the gene. Two copies also means there is an even stronger predisposition to gluten sensitivity than having one gene and the resultant immunologic gluten sensitivity may be more severe."

Interpretation of Fecal Anti-gliadin Antibody: "Intestinal antibody was elevated, indicating that you have active dietary gluten sensitivity. For optimal health, resolution of symptoms and prevention of small intestinal damage and malnutrition, osteoporosis, and damage to other tissues (like nerves, brain, joints, muscles, thyroid, pancreas, other glands, skin, liver, spleen, among others), it is recommended that you follow a strict and permanent gluten-free diet. As gluten sensitivity is a genetic syndrome, you may want to have your relatives screened as well."

Interpretation of Fecal Anti-casein Antibody: "Levels of fecal antibody to a food antigen greater than 10 and indicative of an immune reaction, and hence immunologic 'sensitivity' to that food. For any elevated fecal antibody level, it is recommended to remove that food from your diet. Values less than 10 indicate there currently is minimal or no reaction to that food and hence, no direct evidence of food sensitivity to that specific food. However because 1 in 500 people cannot make antibodies at all, and rarely, some people can still have clinically significant reactions to a food antigen despite the lack of significant antibody reaction (because the reactions primarily involve T cells), if you have an immune syndrome or symptoms associated with food sensitivity, it is recommended that you try a strict removal of suspect foods from your diet for up to 12 months despite a negative test."

These were only a couple of my intolerances that I thankfully found out about when I was tested in October 2008.

Certain immune reactions cannot only cause physiological 'fog,' they can also affect us right down to our second 'brain' which of course is the gut causing physical symptoms. There are so many factors that occur when the digestion system feels compromised. This is an area of study that even the best specialists are learning more and more about. Unfortunately this disease is a huge unknown and there are many different pieces of this complex puzzle still trying to be figured out.

Another health related issue I have to go through and understand is Candida. Additionally there is also Perianal disease. Perianal fistulas and abscesses are serious manifestations of also having Crohn's. Some complications can even lead to difficulties with recurrent or non-healing fistulas/abscesses. Having to learn to live with this also puts a risk of incontinence which could unfortunately result in having severe damage. Going through surgery for my fistula/abscess I was not even aware that I had any major health issues. It was years later when I was finally diagnosed with Crohn's.

Other related symptoms of dealing with Crohn's are spouts of anxiety. Depression alone has many different symptoms and depending on the severity it can be treated differently. Unfortunately no one living with such health complications can eliminate going through the symptoms of anxiety and depression. I was embarrassed that I was dealing with any of it. However after learning that the symptoms in my case where anything from sleep deprivation, lack and change of appetite, feeling agitated, feeling extreme guilt, etc., I was shocked and realized that I had no reason to be embarrassed… only proud of myself for wanting to understand what I needed to learn about myself mentally.

I learned that even as healthy as one can be, you will go through any of these symptoms at one time or another, maybe more, but will probably never have the courage to accept that they need help or be okay with an actual diagnosis of their mental health. However on the upside there are many forms of depression and I am fortunate that most of my symptoms occur depending on how much this disease is controlled – especially as I have learned throughout the past several years. I am not only a product of my environment, but also a product of my parents, and we naturally take on 40% of their immune system. I have learned that hereditarily, psychologically and physically we don't have too much of a choice with what our parents pass down to us. There is no fault or blame either, however there is the truth and we must accept that.

Taking accountability for your overall health is not easy, nor is specifically learning about who we are. I had to learn that some of my past emotional trauma was very much present even though I didn't think about or feel the shame from it. Not having worked through thoughts every way possible allows lingering emotions, and I would wonder at times why I would feel more stress than others. I'd be agitated by others responses, feeling unwell physically, drained emotionally, or feel like my plate was full. I didn't know that we hold on to many hurt emotions and they will play their role when we least expect it. Our subconscious and our present thoughts are very powerful. I had been through therapy and discussed my issues, so I thought from that point I was good to go and I didn't need to work through anything else. I know many people who think the same way and if they seek council a few times it's good enough. What I have learned is this: it takes continual and consistent involvement of showing up emotionally, being vulnerable, and being able to express yourself in a pure and honest way from both your past to the present. Most people I know don't want to relive or talk about the emotional thoughts and feelings whether it be past or present. However through my own personal experience this is key to how we attain ultimate physiological health. Daring to show up for our emotional health once a month even, and use that time for your very personal thoughts and feelings, in my experience empowers the purpose and reminds me of who I am. Even if we are embarrassed or feel shame from something in our past, in my experience it is our responsibility to resolve these issues.

Living with anxiety and learning how to get certain chemical release into the body is very important – and not only for those living with more health complications – because this is a natural process every human has and goes through. This ranges from secretion of hormones or chemicals to taking in the proper nutrition, exercise, and of course having a good environmental structure. From my experience it can make a significant difference in the way one feels and thinks. I have seen a lot of people who mask their symptoms and just go through everyday life with whatever it takes to get through that day or week. Whether it be certain prescribed medications or over the counter drugs, many daily caffeinated beverages, excess sugars, overconsumption of carbohydrates, and/or even starvation. Taking accountability on every cellular level in my experience is a full-time job and then some. It is being accountable 24/7 and you don't get to have a day 'off,' but it is a choice you make.

Sadly, I feel that too many times it may come across or be interpreted that I do not have any real kind of control with this disease, or that it is an emotional state of being that is consistently making me hide behind the diagnosis of Crohn's. That being said, it is very complicated and a lot of what I have described is merely a preview of my daily life when trying to describe some of it. I am also someone who has chosen a more natural approach, and in doing so understanding that managing my symptoms, nutrition and lifestyle is by far the hardest course of action to take. Naturally at this point in my healing and living with my IBD which is still not fully in remission, I also had to learn about my own personal behaviours – how they were created and affecting my choices and decisions as a person. Acknowledging personal triggers, addictions, and how they were ultimately affecting my life and my health. I have lost some of my closest friends or our closeness simply because I have changed throughout this process both emotionally and physically. I have made decisions about my health that they either didn't try to understand or agree with the way I have been trying to heal. Not caring about what people think is one of the hardest lessons I have had to go through in this journey, and to this day I still struggle with it at times. Some assume that if I just have surgery or take some medication all the pain will go away and I can start from scratch. Either that or I will hopefully stop complaining and venting about the pain or struggles that I go through. Most people unfortunately feel that way because I live on full-time disability and I must have a great life being 'off' work and enjoying all this free time on my hands. What an arrogant way to think, and at times it has got my blood boiling!

Most people make comments and offer their assumed wanted advice without having much knowledge or experience with what it is they are commenting on. I do understand that when you love someone and make an assumption it is naturally because it is difficult to hear and see them in pain, especially when it comes from my family. Over the years this has become somewhat frustrating at times as I work so hard on my health and they just don't get it or try to understand what it actually entails. I won't get asked too much about the specifics regarding what it is I am really trying to do. At times it can feel like the carpet is being pulled out from under me, and anything I say or explain goes in one ear and out the other. It is as though I must not really know what I am doing because I am still 'sick,' when in fact I have come so far and my medical and therapeutic team around me are amazed with what I am able to do and how I take care of this condition.

I don't know exactly what I would tell my good friend if I had to continue to hear about how they were being affected by an illness. What I can say now, having lived through this journey, is so far as denying surgery and drugs at this point in my life: if you can find ways to manage any of the pain with accountability, hard work, sacrifice, dedication and be able to find the support in believing that you are worth the best care possible, then what you feel you can do is going to be the best choice and decision that you can make. No one else can make these decisions for you even if they are the best doctor. You alone have to make the choice before anyone can help lead you. It is not easy by any means to find amazing doctors or have a work environment that will even allow you the time off while not threatening your job... yet at the same time supporting what you are choosing to do as well as those opinions and recommendations of your doctors. That is such a huge part of the healing process and I understand that better than most, especially after what I have been through, that it is possible.

Adding another medical doctor to my team, which I had been wanting to do for a very long time, was a General Practitioner (GP). I had never had a female GP before as an adult and felt blessed to have her accept me as one of her patients. I had my very first physical appointment in September 2010. She was great, extremely thorough, and continues to impress me whenever I see her. It was also nice to get away from the gynecologist who I had been seeing for the past couple of years. Unfortunately almost every appointment had been a little stressful even though she was a specialist in the field. I had been referred to her because of a number of concerns from my past... mostly having abnormal cells.

Dr. C. is my main doctor and teaches me his own insightful wisdom, including the root causes of living with an inflammatory bowel disease, having food intolerances, and living with Candida. I also needed a family doctor who could advise me medically, do my yearly physicals, blood work, drug prescriptions and medical referrals. Naturally she would also be copied on work done by my other doctors and specialists. I really liked this GP and loved her approach. Her personality and empathy allowed me to trust her right away. I am very lucky indeed.

Discussed initially with Dr. C., he thought it was time for me to see another GE specialist as it had been a year and a half since my last GE. Even though Dr. C. was now my main doctor and doing all the communication with my insurance company, having a GE while going through IBD is important. I was also going through yearly and quarterly medical evaluations with my insurance company, as well as dealing with an evaluation to apply for CPP disability benefits which the insurance company insisted I do. The medical team at my insurance company also felt that even though my doctor was providing exceptional medical feedback and I was showing progress, that an opinion from a GE specialist was still needed since I was going through this evaluation process. It is understandable considering that every patient living with an inflammatory bowel disease has a GE specialist who does the initial diagnosis. My insurance company wanted me to see their doctors for evaluations, namely a psychologist and a GE specialist. I met with their psychologist for evaluation. Unfortunately the GE they wanted me to see was too far away for me to get to, but soon thereafter I was referred to a GE specialist by Dr. C. and my GP. I met with him in the early spring of April 2011.

With everything I had going on and just trying to get through my days with managing my symptoms, I wasn't able to meet anyone's expectations and felt it was best to stop my studies through the online courses I was taking.

Chapter 7

Changing Definition of Disability

The recommendations and opinions from doctors and GE specialists were very important to have for the medical board at my insurance company. Even more so when trying to have my full-time disability status approved. Normally working with a new physician, especially a gastroenterologist specialist, requires redoing blood work, CT scans, an MRI exam, and of course having another colonoscopy.

I was anxious to meet this new GE specialist because I was scared of what he was going to say. I was scared about what he was going think of how I had been healing without opting for surgery or taking medications. I was worried about what he was going to ask me to do or what treatment he felt was best for me to pursue. I had started this new journey with Dr. C. and it felt right. I felt supported and properly guided in learning about my health overall. I was learning about what foods were triggering my immune system and why. Even though I was trying so hard, nutrition was merely one aspect adding havoc to my immune system which caused my body to defend itself. Dr. C. calls it as it is, a puzzle.

With having Crohn's and facing higher levels of inflammation, which was being measured through examinations and blood work, part of what this disease does is it won't allow for complete nutrient absorption. This is partly because Crohn's affects the intestine and usually the small bowel area where people without IBD absorb many of their key nutrients. Many of the body's nutrients are absorbed in the gut and intestines. Since Crohn's affects a portion of the intestines, it doesn't allow for complete nutrient absorption, period. It's a lot harder for me to get the vitamins and minerals the body needs to be healthy and repair itself when it isn't getting enough absorbed and its energy is already being used by the illness. For me, having to adhere to a very restricted diet makes it one tough game.

I was still going through a lot of pain while eating certain foods, feeling overwhelmed, and most often feeling stressed out not knowing exactly why or what was going on. Sometimes I would be fine after eating something. Other times after eating I'd experience some pain to feeling the worst kind of pain due to what seemed to be the smallest simplest thing. This merry-go-round seemed never-ending.

I was grateful to have my husband with me during the initial appointment with my second gastroenterologist specialist. To my surprise he was quite gentle in his approach. He was very experienced and took the time to listen and was quite empathetic. He reviewed my previous tests and procedures. The most recent exam that I had just been through was an ultrasound which he noted showed an improvement. He wanted me to go through more testing and procedures. I explained with worry that I had gone through a rough first colonoscopy and was not ready to go through that procedure again. I also explained that I had recently gone through a CT scan and wanted to stay away from radiation at this time if possible. He recommended that I have an MRI and bloodwork. He also recommended that I not return to my position at work and continue to work on my health full-time. He understood how time consuming it was to try living with and attempt healing with active Crohn's as naturally as I could. He knew that just learning to live with the disease, keeping my mental status in check on a daily basis, and following a recommended diet to maintain the daily symptoms while trying to have decent energy was more than enough to deal with and would continue to be a full-time job. He expressed that he believed I was on the right path and would also support the hard discipline and routine that I have had to incorporate into my everyday life. What was really a shock to hear was that through this healing process he suggested trying to enjoy my life while continuing to learn how to live with my illness. Coming from a GE that made me feel supported and happy with my choices thus far. He also recommended that I try a mild drug to be taken daily called Pentasa which apparently works well in the small intestine specifically, while helping to keep inflammation down and give my intestine a little time to rest, hoping that things wouldn't get worse. He said he would send his notes of our appointment and his recommendations to Dr. C. With a follow-up appointment in six months, I left his office feeling good about our appointment and a prescription for Pentasa.

I was continuing to reduce the amount of gluten, dairy and processed sugars in my diet as well as the other foods, beverages, additives and preservatives that were causing immune reactions. Having tried this new approach for a couple of years, I felt okay most days but continued to struggle through the other days as though pain was a normal part of my everyday life. The struggle to know exactly what was causing me to get sick so quickly some days and not the others, I can only describe as one of the biggest stressors of this disease. While I was getting my nutrition under control and trying to remove additional environmental stressors, changing behaviours, daily routine, perspective and learning to change the way I even looked at nutrition was and continues to be an everyday battle. Additionally there was other pain that I suffered that was still creating a load of stress for me. However this pain was emotional. Stress is one of the biggest triggers for anyone's health. When living with a chronic inflammatory condition it takes an even greater toll on your body and your health. Stress from sugar contributes to damaging body cells, killing off good bacteria, changing the gut flora and contributes to causing flare-ups in the body. These are unfortunately only a few damaging health issues that happen to the immune system when inflammation is triggered. There is also an emotional connection to physical symptoms. Having an open mind and the courage to take in the emotional awareness helped me understand and want even greater overall health, as well as a stronger platform to feel and walk from. Having to link my emotions psychologically with my 'second brain,' the gut, has taken accountability, insight, great awareness, willpower and the experience of living with an inflammatory bowel disease. I have been very fortunate to not only learn about the connection between the two, but also my daily structure is set up to embrace the continual balance of learning from them.

Now for a little of my personal history: I was born the 5th child with a smile, as my mother would say, and weighed in at approximately 7 pounds 9 ounces. Unfortunately it wasn't until much later in my life that I learned about having a weakened immune system, and also what my mother described as being raised in somewhat of a stressful environment. My parents are both very strong, loving people, and growing up they did what they could with what they knew and had. To this day either one of them would give me the shirt off their back and their last dollar if needed. When I close my eyes and try to go back to those very early years I am left with minimal memory. I have senses of certain memories, whether it be an old piece of clothing or a smell, and these memories sometimes sit in my mind with a hint of once knowing and experiencing in my past. From what I have always been told about those times in my life, I was a happy kid. I smiled a lot, always wanting to have fun and play sports. My siblings say they cared for me often and that I wasn't difficult to deal with, most often anyways. Sometimes I wish I could remember my younger days as they claim they do. Only until recently have I been able to link the emotional scarring that this held over me. Being born the youngest of five, later on I realized that this was going to be one of the biggest challenges of my life to overcome.

Being the youngest of five I always had my three sisters, brother, their friends and our extended family around. All through middle school and high school, I had enough friends which I felt good about most days. Looking back however I didn't always fit in, feel special or have the self-esteem of feeling good enough on a consistent basis. Having older siblings, I was always faced with comparing myself to them or having my parents, family, whomever, compare each of us to each other. Surely this was innocent at the time, however wanting to be like someone else or being compared too much, I can personally say starts at a very young age and didn't help me feel confident in who I was. It became normal to seek the approval of others before my own. For those like me out there who come from a big family, I am sure you can relate.

Being the youngest I had a lot of opinions around me. Do's and don'ts thrown at me and until recently, I didn't know any better or any different. I was always told to go with this sister or that one, it didn't matter what they were doing either. I idolized my sisters and acted like them as much as I could. They were always the coolest! Now being an adult, taking care of my own affairs and having the opportunity to learn about myself, I feel that much of that admiration to want to be like them enabled behaviours of wanting and needing to be like others before being okay with who I was. Needing and seeking the approval of others, or caring too much about what other people thought, also enabled an insecure behaviour of needing the acceptance and approval of others in some way. Speaking from my own experience and sharing with many others over time, I realize that I was not alone in feeling this way. We are all seeking love and approval. We all need love and want to feel loved. We all need affection. We all want to feel accepted and acknowledged for our efforts or accomplishments. The most important platform that I have learned to work on is the relationship you have with yourself. If you do not love and accept yourself, how can you ask anyone else to love you?

Finally, after fearing the worst and dealing with everything inside me to keep positive and trust in the journey I was on, things were about to change. At the end of June 2011 I received another letter from my insurance company. It stated: "Your claim for long-term disability benefits has been accepted beyond the 24-month decision point. Our letter of April 2011 discussed the change in definition of disability." My full-time disability had been approved, and I knew in that moment that everything was happening for a reason. I finally felt a little more secure with what I was doing and was able to have good faith in my insurance company. Even more so because they had also given me another case worker who I was beyond happy with and more than grateful to have managing my case. In the beginning I was someone who was fighting to return to work, and it took a lot for me to even consider taking any time off… let alone now being happy in having my health become my full-time job.

Having received the good news from my insurance company was a blessing. What came next soon thereafter, in my opinion, was a sign of being watched over in some spiritual way. Like I said and believe, things happen for many reasons, and I'm just not sure if we get the chance to always know why when we need to.

After seeing Dr. C. and going over the notes of my GE from my appointment earlier that April, he was also concerned that my liver enzymes were not where they needed to be. I left with a requisition for blood work and a request for an MRI that my GE had also recommended. I hoped to have the MRI done before my next scheduled appointment with my GE, which was in August, so we'd be able to go over the results right away.

Soon after my appointment with Dr. C. I started to experience similar pain to that when I had initially been very ill and couldn't get out of bed. My symptoms got progressively worse the week after receiving the news from my insurance company. I felt my body getting more tired and weak. My cramps and contractions went from moderate to severe. Things felt different and I wasn't able to get out of bed for literally two weeks. To the day, it was fifteen days of lying in bed. I could barely make it to the washroom and had several accidents in bed and on our new king sized mattress. Some nights were so rough that thankfully my husband would check on me during the late night and find me sweating, almost fainting in the bathroom on the floor. He'd sit with me and be by my side, waiting and trying to remain patient while I could find the strength to get up. It was then that I had some of the scariest moments of my life and I wasn't sure how things were going to progress. At times I would even think to myself, is this it? My husband would help me get the sheets off the bed that had diarrhea on them. It was so embarrassing having him deal with the foul smell of it all, especially being all hours of the night and having to wake up from your sleep to deal with such a situation. Feeling completely mortified at what was going on, my husband simply loved me through every step and took amazing care of me. I will never forget what he has done for me, nor how he has continued to love and support me more and more with every passing day.

I slowly got back on my feet, and had never felt so thankful. Simply having the energy to get up and walk to another room felt amazing. I was very cautious about what I would eat, other than broth, toast, potatoes or the odd Popsicle to suck on. I was scared to eat, and it also felt like my stomach had just undergone surgery and was very sensitive.

It wasn't before too long that I was heading into my appointment to have an MRI. It was scheduled right before the next meeting with my GE, which was just in time. I was pretty nervous as I really do not like being in a hospital or having to get an IV. Due to the fact that they needed a certain test done, I was required to have injections while in the MRI machine. The tech 'botched' my IV and made me bleed while I had to keep in the catheter. I also learned that the injections were done by a machine, so I would have to keep my arms out in front of me while lying on my stomach going through the MRI scan.

I met my GE the following day, anxious to know the results. These MRI results were being compared to the earlier MRI done in November 2008. As it showed, I went through a high grade obstruction. Here are the details from the MRI scan: "The most striking findings on today's examination is the presence of the marked small bowel dilatation. Most of the abdominal pelvic recesses are occupied by distended bowel loops. The caliber of the maximally distended loop measures in the order of 5.7 cm. It is difficult to decipher the transition point. The large bowel is of normal caliber. No appreciable bowel wall thickening is identified. Bowel wall enhancement is unremarkable. There is no interloop abscess. Previously documented heterogeneous areas along the sub capsular aspect of the hepatic dome are no longer identifiable. There is no hepatomegaly either. Please note, however, that the study was not tailored to evaluate the liver. No worrisome focal liver lesions. No intra-/extra hepatic biliary dilatation. Conclusion: Marked dilatation of the small bowel with collapse of the large bowel is consistent with high grade obstruction. Bowel wall enhancement is within normal limits. It is difficult to decipher the exact location of the transition point. I suspect there is likely a stricture at the level of the distal and terminal ileum, though this cannot be confirmed due to limited spatial resolution and marked bowel distension with its associated mass effect on adjacent structures. No focal or diffuse liver abnormality is identified within the limitations of the current study. The patient may benefit from a CT enterography in the future given its improved spatial resolution."

It also showed that I had additional pressure from inflammation in the ileocecal valve. Attached to the ileocecal valve is the ileum area – being the last part of the small intestine – which is where my actual 'diseased bowel' is located.

I explained honestly that I had not taken any of the Pentasa medication. In detail I explained what I had also just gone through – being so ill and in bed for two weeks. Due to how severe things were and how I was feeling, with a firm tone he suggested steroids right away. He wanted a stronger steroid because he wasn't sure if Pentasa would even make enough of a difference at this point. He also recommended that I stick with only fluids until the symptoms subsided. I left his office with another steroid prescription and started Pentasa that afternoon.

Feeling absolutely terrified that I was headed for emergency surgery and harsher steroids, soon afterwards I had a conversation with Dr. C. and he also felt that the only way I could continue healing without surgery at that point was to go on steroids for a short while, hoping it would help calm my small bowel. He recommended that without having surgery, learning to incorporate my nutrition with mostly liquids and a low residue diet would be the best way for me to continue on as my bowel was in a severe state. This would not only allow me to absorb nutrition better, but also allow the obstructed area to digest more easily and cause less pain while processing food. As a section of my bowel was now obstructed, as well as very narrow and filled with scar tissue, I was in a place where other than hoping the steroids would give me some relief to avoid emergency surgery, there were minimal options. They described my obstructed area as being similar to the size of a straw that was being put into a balloon that was only half blown up. While other segments of the intestines are the width of a banana-sized straw, the obstructed section didn't give me

85

a lot of room to have solids go through. I was scared at this point of potentially having a perforation of the bowel, which would definitely lead to emergency surgery and further complications.

Dr. C. followed up with my GE immediately, and between the two of them they were okay with me starting with a fluid diet, then incorporating a pureed low residue liquid diet. Dr. C. left me with solid advice and sent me information to begin with the diet.

From August 25th, 2011, onwards, my choices, values, perspectives, nutrition and everyday life changed.

Chapter 8

What Did It Take to Live on Liquids?

After learning about the obstruction results, I then had a very heartfelt and teary-eyed conversation with Dr. C., feeling terrified more so than ever. Our time together somehow helped me have enough desire for the 'want' in choosing better for my health and overall self from that moment on. I wanted to be better and do better for myself. I had been given a beautiful opportunity, having time on my side and great support to try and heal. What's more, I also wanted to learn to try and cope with this condition.

Learning to feel good enough and confident in making choices has taught me many things. Learning proper discipline and what you may have to sacrifice to achieve results have been huge lessons, even today. I have learned patience and compassion while facing my fears, shame, anxiety and guilt. One of the hardest forms of therapy in which I continue to work at is retraining my brain, while also focusing diligently to unlearn certain learned behaviours. In changing into who I want to be, finding the strength everyday has been and continues to be a journey in itself.

The very next day after seeing my GE and getting on a plan with him and Dr. C., I had started to live solely on liquids. To help settle the obstructed area and inflammation I began with nutritional shakes for three months. Then I started to incorporate my own smoothie blends, juicing blends and puree soups. I was on a completely liquid diet for six months and never went off course, but my nutrition was extremely limited. After feeling a lot better eggs became such a treat because I had missed chewing so much, and they became a big part of my everyday protein. I can only describe my willpower and determination with simply accepting that: 1) I had no real option other than surgery which could lead to other potential complications, and 2) my obstructed intestines were worth it. I had to dig deep every minute of the day. I didn't have much energy or time for anything or anyone other than focusing on what that day brought. I had to learn to be in the moment and simply learn to feel just that.

To help get through the cravings for solid food, chewing, and also salivating while others ate around me or going over the amount of liquid I was taking, I was fortunate to have the love and support of my husband who has always been by my side. As well, I focused on putting together a 2,000-piece puzzle. This puzzle has become a framed piece and is a constant reminder of those times. Sitting every day in silence so that I could focus solely on that made it possible for me to even attempt what seemed like an impossible diet. It took weeks to get into a routine with liquids and it wasn't easy. At the time my stomach had gone through so much pain that I was terrified to even attempt eating solids. Mentally, I was ready to change, and this was the beginning of my transformation. This was how my discipline began. Was it hard core? Absolutely. Did I have to learn a great deal about patience? You bet. I learned how to retrain my thoughts around nutrition and finally understood how the smallest thing could have an effect on symptoms. I realized that if I didn't put 100% of my energy towards dealing with this condition and with my overall health, then my future was going to be at risk.

After working my way through cravings and accepting that while for most people having a smoothie for all meals seemed crazy, one of the hardest things was trying to make those in my life understand why I was doing it. Or trying to get them to understand why I couldn't go to a special occasion or just come over for a little visit… even spending time with family or just meeting up at a restaurant for tea. I was focused on forgetting about almost everything to do with the regular way people celebrate with food. Every occasion was something different, but always went back to having some kind of food. One of the hardest issues to deal with while going through my healing has been losing some of my best friends. I was on a mission, one of a lonely pilgrim. By choice, yes, but a lonely one nonetheless. I lost friendships that I thought were unbreakable, and I had many hurt feelings that at times I thought for sure I would give into temptations. I felt judged at times and misunderstood by most of those in my life. I found it very difficult to relate to anyone with the day-to-day happenings of life. Even now my friends and family progress in their accomplishments, but I get very little acknowledgment about mine. Working towards a routine and trying to manage my symptoms, I needed to stay in my zone and conserve my energy for my own well-being.

I didn't do this just because I wanted to be alone or difficult, but instead I was trying to put a very serious health condition into remission. I still am.

Immediately after learning about my obstruction my osteopath worked on my body, which has always helped my entire body feel much better. I can't express enough how amazing this woman's therapy is and how having her friendship has inspired me. Together we even came up with affirmations that would also help change my brain matter. They helped reinforce my wandering thoughts to those of having strong will, good discipline, encouragement and love. Taking the next 365 days to simply incorporate a new way of being, thinking and changing, I didn't miss one session with myself. I would do this regiment in the mornings to begin my day with gratefulness, strength, guidance and compassion for the way I was choosing to heal. My doctors also recommended that I also try doing a form of exercise on a daily basis to help both physically and mentally.

As time passed my everyday regiment became more and more of a routine. I began to flourish in my nutrition even though it continued to be very strict. I developed a schedule that allowed proper prep time for the nutrition I needed. I made my spiritual, mental and physical self accountable. I had a team of doctors and therapists who I worked with on a daily, weekly and monthly basis. I began to create healthy boundaries with my energy and how much time I could give another person. I gave myself time when I needed to simply rest and be with whatever symptom I would be feeling. In my experience no transition happens overnight. Working away and being present every day while keeping a daily dedicated routine was the only way that I could feel as though what I was doing really mattered. After almost two years this was no longer just an everyday routine. This was my lifestyle. A lifestyle created to manage and maintain a very difficult, almost unmanageable, full-time condition. This became my full-time job.

I have been documenting my everyday life since being on full-time disability in the fall of 2008. In August 2017 it will be six years since my transition truly began, and it has been quite the journey.

On November 21st, 2013, I met Dr. O. She was my third GE specialist since I was originally diagnosed with Crohn's in the winter of 2006. I was fine with the GE I had been seeing and working with, however he was no longer in the hospital and was moving towards the last stages of his career. We had discussed having me meet this new GE specialist, and I was pleased since I had always wanted a female GE. There are few women specialists in this field, and I had not heard of one taking new patients up until this point. He was very honest with me and said that this GE in particular was great and would be a very good fit for me, especially going into the future. He made the request to her office.

To be honest I was a little afraid and very anxious to hear her thoughts and opinions. After meeting with her, however, I left her office feeling understood and more supported than my previous two GE specialists. Being a new patient though, she wanted me to go through new blood work, an MRI, a CT scan, and a colonoscopy.

I was very fearful and had a lot of anxiety just thinking about how painful the colonoscopy procedure was going to be this time around. I was afraid about how much sedation and the amount of gas that would be used. I was nervous wondering if she was even going to be able to get into the stricture as discussed, or how much pain that would potentially cause. We discussed that most of the pain would depend on what space she could move through with the scope once entering the ileum area. She explained about possibly trying a balloon-like instrument that could be expanded inside to help make that obstructed area wider. This could possibly allow me to process things a little less painfully if we could do it. This was the goal. However the small section of the ileocecal valve from my last MRI showed that inflammation was adding pressure in that valve area already. Naturally I was worried about the pain this procedure was going to cause.

Before long it was time to begin the prep work for this procedure. Looking back at my first colonoscopy seven years ago and the preparation for it, I felt that this time around was already a much different experience. In preparing for this colonoscopy, the osteopath whom I had been seeing religiously every month since 2009 worked on my body and specifically in my anus to relieve tight muscles and help relax the area during the procedure. Having had a couple rectal exams in my life, this is one treatment that I would recommend to anyone if you're ever scheduled to have one done. This is one of the steps that should be an option when having a colonoscopy.

With my nerves being at an all-time high, adding the pain of my PMS and beginning the process for the preparation of the colonoscopy procedure was rough. In having to take tablets of Bisacodyl (which is a stimulant laxative) as well Pico-Salax, I made sure to put a long towel down before falling asleep that night, just in case.

The laxatives made me feel very nauseous, and going from one bowel movement to another my bum was starting to feel raw. Drained from worrying and thinking about how everything was going to go, I just kept telling myself it's going to be okay, it's going to be okay.

The second night of preparation didn't go so well. The laxatives started off with having mild to moderate cramping, and I was nauseous and had minimal energy. I thought I was through the worst of it, how naïve. Not only was I starving and visualized myself eating everything possible, the knot feeling of 'nasty' was now getting stronger. The main ingredient in the Pico-Salax was citric acid. This ingredient is derived from yeast. Additives and preservatives can disrupt the friendly bacteria and allow the yeast to flourish. Being that I already suffer with having yeast issues, it seemed that this ingredient just killed my stomach. I was in sweats by 11:00 pm, down on my knees in front of the toilet praying that I would be okay. I have never actually fainted, came very close at times, but literally thought it was going to happen because I felt so sick.

Going through this painful preparation, I was very grateful to have my husband close by that evening because being in that amount of pain and scared to faint, I couldn't speak and even worse could barely move.

Having him beside me and just being present was a huge comfort.

The following morning, which was the morning of the exam, I was having bowel contraction cramping and binding pain from my bowels. I was not feeling well at all. On top of that I was now bleeding from having started my period, and thought, hopefully I don't cause too much of a mess during my exam. My last bowel movement was around 6:00 am, and I was not allowed to drink any more fluids until after my procedure. We arrived at the hospital by 10:30 am, and my procedure started around 12:30 pm. This time was different in a few ways, starting with the fact that I was in a bed to receive my IV. A nurse went through a list of questions, and I was in a recovery ward watching others come out of their sedation. I laid there in the recovery unit waiting until the actual procedure took place. My husband wasn't allowed to sit with me, which definitely would have helped calm my nerves. It was my turn for the procedure at 12:50 pm. I was wheeled on the bed into the procedure room. Dr. O. came in minutes later and I asked her if I could have half the sedation amount because I was terribly sick the night prior with the preparation. I was afraid of being too sedated and feeling more nauseous. I would rather feel the uncomfortable pain of the scope. She agreed.

As she slowly entered the scope it was actually tolerable. Wheef! Usually anything entering the rectum is quite awful, however the osteopathy work from my therapist that I just had a week prior really seemed to help.

There I was lying on my left side with an IV in my right arm. After receiving the injection of fentanyl and IV Diazemuls, I felt like I had just been given a shot of morphine. I felt very heavy in the head. It lasted for about 2 to 5 minutes, but then thankfully I was feeling better and was more consciously aware of the actual procedure. Watching the scope moving down the large colon, watching the blood from the biopsies get flushed away as she cut them off my intestinal linings, it didn't feel too painful but I could definitely feel it. She was able to get right down past the ileocecal value/cecum into my ileum area, where my actual 'diseased bowel' is. It was weird to see how 'caved in looking' my small intestine looked with the obstructed blown out section compared to the large intestine. (This was how they described the straw-like size going into a balloon shape.) It was definitely painful at that point and thankfully she didn't spend too much time there, but she was able to at least see what was going on. Withdrawing the instrument from inside me and the rectal exam at the end of the procedure felt a little uncomfortable, but I tolerated it well.

When I heard the magical words, "All finished, you can now go into recovery," what a relief I felt, and into the recovery room I went.

I waited in the recovery room for about an hour and felt better than expected. All I wanted to do was get the IV out of my arm and see my husband. Finally I was able to leave and my husband took me home.

Back home, having started my period and now dealing with a little blood in my stool from the procedure, I felt a little like a bloody mess. I was ready to get my comfortable clothes on and get all snuggled up and eat! This time around however a big treat for me was a bowl of garlic mashed potatoes that my husband made for me.

In having any procedure there is, of course, the waiting to find out the results. I was also waiting to have my MRI exam as I still had two exams to go. I finally confirmed it was scheduled for the end of January 2014. My GE wanted a comparison to my MRI exam from August 2011, which indicated: "Dilatation of the small bowel and collapse of the large bowel is consistent with high grade obstruction. A stricture at the level of the distal and terminal ileum. Marked bowel distension with its associated mass effect on adjacent structures." As well, my MRI from April 2013 showed that there was some distension of the cecum and colon. There was also some prestenotic dilation of the small bowel. I also had mild intrahepatic bile duct dilation with slight irregularity – this questioned whether I had primary sclerosing cholangitis.

I was anxious to find out what was going to come from this next MRI.

My final CT enterography exam was scheduled for the middle of February 2014. I knew that I had to have this exam to know exactly what was going on in my abdomen and pelvis, so I was very anxious to have the test over and down with.

While waiting for my next visit with my GE to go over the results from the three exams, I had enough going on in my thoughts that sometimes I would wonder what is wrong with me. Why am I so nervous? I have spent much time worrying about: What's going to happen? With each exam, which tech or nurse will I get? Is it going to hurt? How long is it really going to take? Will I be okay? What is my specialist going to say? What will he/she think of me while reviewing my results? Will they approve of the way I have chosen to heal this far? I am exhausted just thinking about it. I have literally wasted many precious moments, worrying!

At the end of March 2014, it was finally time to go over the results with my GE. She was detailed when explaining my procedure. This is, for the most part, what I was told: "There was no inflammation seen and the vascular pattern was normal from the cecum to the anal verge. Biopsies were taken from the terminal ileum, right colon, left colon, and rectum. There were no polyps or masses seen as we removed the colonoscope. There were no diverticuli. There were no angiodysplastic lesions. There were no hemorrhoids on retroflex view and no other abnormalities." This time my colonoscopy was actually almost normal. It is possible that they did not reach the area that has been strictured in the past. In summary, I was a 32-year-old female with terminal ileal Crohn's disease and probable primary sclerosing cholangitis (PSC).

Having gone through the MRI exam and going over those results, it also showed that I have in fact two intrahepatic duct strictures without significant dilation and this was thought to be consistent with early primary sclerosing cholangitis. I also had hepatimegaly which was unchanged from previous. My liver enzymes were completely normal which was a great sign, however with the PSC diagnosis, I was then referred to a liver specialist. After meeting with the liver specialist she felt that because my enzymes were normal and the strictures were minimal, that having an MRI yearly to monitor would be sufficient.

Lastly, the CT enterography was compared to the previous CT from November 2008. This present exam showed a 17 cm stricture in the ileum with significant dilation of the small bowel proximal to that. There was also an active Crohn's segment that measured 5 cm in the distal ileum. This was considered to be a separate area. Clearly both these areas are proximal to the reach of the scope.

From my initial colonoscopy exam in 2006, it stated that biopsies of the terminal ileum confirmed mild acute and chronic inflammation consistent with Crohn's disease. Having also a small bowel follow through at the time suggested a 20 cm of terminal ileum stricture with some prestenotic dilatation.

Going over the results together with my GE was good and bad. She feels that I will eventually have to have surgery and really can't believe I haven't already because my obstruction area is in too much of an emergency state as is. She feels that in waiting I could end up going through a perforated bowel situation or another obstruction that would force me into an emergency surgery which is something that should be avoided at all costs.

Her recommendations for treatment and follow-up gave me a few choices. One option is to continue with what I am doing now, knowing that I can and will likely develop complications in the future which would include worsening obstruction and potential fistula formation or abscess development. The second option is to see a surgeon now and consider an ileal resection. She thinks I have significant symptoms and am quite limited by my diet, therefore I will likely be a candidate for surgery. The third option is to try prescribed medical therapy which would likely be Imuran with or without Entocort temporarily for induction. This option would potentially delay surgery but would likely not totally prevent it. At the very least it would hopefully decrease the inflammatory segment. We had a long discussion regarding the different options. My GE was okay with my decision to continue doing what I was doing full-time, and suggested that I think about everything we had discussed during our appointment.

My GE noted: I continue to have obstruction symptoms but manage them very well with dietary manipulation. Whenever I have abdominal pain I go on a liquid diet for a while. My diet is very limited. Most of my diet is pureed. Although it appears to be very difficult, I actually seem to be managing this quite well and am happy with the current therapy that I have been doing. I remain on no medications for Crohn's disease.

Also noted was that I do not have any significant colonic disease, therefore I am at average risk for colon cancer. The primary sclerosing cholangitis, as far as she knows, should not increase my risk of colon cancer in the absence of colonic disease. She would recommend, to be on the safe side, surveillance colonoscopies once every five years.

We left her office feeling relieved with some of the information, yet still had remaining worries for the others.

I usually go through waves of emotion after leaving an appointment. There was a lot to take in, and sometimes it all feels surreal that I am even dealing with any of it. On one hand I feel grateful to have a great specialist like her and I am hopeful she will be my GE for as long as I need her. I am grateful to learn about what is actually going on with my health and feel my GE uses language I can understand. I am grateful that I don't feel too much pressure to heal in one specific way as I have in the past. I also feel grateful to have her support and that of my entire medical team, as well as the select few people in my life who have been part of this journey.

Yet on the other hand, when thinking about what treatment or avenue to choose there are unfortunately no guarantees. With having surgery there are many complications that could arise. Or worse, set me up for having more surgeries down the road. Taking medications which would suppress the immune system and help with keeping inflammation controlled can also lead to many side effects. Having the 'what ifs' or 'what should I do' have been and continue to always be on my mind.

In the beginning I was terrified to think about having surgery, it shook me to my core. Over the years of battling through this fear I understand why it is recommended and why most people with IBD have it right away. I have also heard and read about many people who are in a worse place because they had surgery. In my particular situation my GE believes I would do well and there is a chance that I would never have to have another re-section. Every year I learn more. Having been on steroids three times has already turned me off from wanting to be on daily medication. Now I am getting to the point where I am thinking of booking an appointment with a surgeon to also hear their perspective because I have questions and concerns that my GE recommends that I ask, specifically with the obstructed areas and the additional 5 cm. This segment of bowel is adding pressure on other areas of the intestines potentially above it, and this would be something that a surgeon would hopefully have more insight and knowledge about. Surgery doesn't feel like the answer for me, however I do not want to end up in an emergency situation either. Information is knowledge. In the future I will hear what advice and opinion a surgeon would have to offer.

I now see my GE specialist every six months and have been building a very good relationship with her. She is not only very kind and considerate but also empathetic, which I find is rare with doctors. She is thorough and I have become very comfortable with her. I feel very supported, acknowledged and always leave our meetings with solid advice and options that I understand. I feel very lucky to have her as my gastroenterologist specialist.

Chapter 9

Life Has Many Surprises

Approaching May 2014 seemed to be coming in with waves of feeling good most days and others having to be still and patient with my symptoms. It will be seven years that I have been working with my health full-time. At times it still feels as though it was only yesterday that I first received the diagnosis of Crohn's, the turning point in my life where I had to accept the fact that in some ways I was simply different. In other ways I feel blessed with how much I have been able to learn and experience in the journey that I have been on. In my experience, going through physical and emotional pain can cause such distress and make it seem impossible to continue on with any real sense of motivation or have any kind of happy life. While I would continue to step back into the ring while feeling like I had lost all control after not feeling well, I began to learn that showing up at all was half the battle. My husband, team of doctors and therapists would remind me of just that.

Mother's Day was approaching that weekend and my loving husband had always made an effort to acknowledge my 'mother-ness' to our little dog, Guinness. He was such a part of us that he truly felt like our baby.

Through the past weeks I had been going through a very tired and draining time. My stomach felt completely off and it was very difficult to try and explain how I felt inside.

One morning that week I remember holding Guinness and thinking, how could I be so tired. I was worried something else was wrong with me. I began to stress about what else I was going to have to deal with. Little did I know, I was actually pregnant!

I will never forget that Mother's Day because I was in complete shock about being pregnant. Also not long thereafter we sadly lost our beloved Guinness, who meant everything to us. We were completely heartbroken. Even now that it has been a year later we always think of him and his perfect little self every day.

Knowing that I now had something very important happening inside of me, I had to bring this news to my doctors and therapists. I was in disbelief and scared. This seemed impossible as I had only been off birth control for a few weeks. Of course knowing that there is always that possibility, my reasoning for getting off the pill was for medical concerns.

Learning the following week from my GP, after taking an official urine test, I was in fact 4 to 6 weeks pregnant. And just like that the journey of motherhood began.

I can tell you from my own experience that I had no choice but to have a high risk obstetrician (OB) to take care of my pregnancy. My GP referred me to one female doctor who had a great reputation and was well experienced in the field. At the time, however, I wanted to do my own research and try to find someone else. I had read her reviews online and although there were good ones, there were ones that I didn't really like. I began to research a few high risk OB's, however two of the three rejected me... I felt not only because I had Crohn's, but also because my baby was due December 31st. Even though I tried not to take it too personally, I do understand why some doctors would not want to add that to their plate. I attempted to get a midwife but the company I had called didn't return my call until weeks later, and at that point I was already working with my OB. The last feeling I wanted to have was: who is going to take care of us?

I decided to withhold my judgment and went in to meet with the first OB who was referred by my GP. All I can say is that I am very glad I did. We got along very well and I felt confident with having her care. We saw each other every month, and every appointment went well. My ultrasounds were great and the first three months were just fine.

From the moment I learned I was pregnant, I had also reached out to my GE to ask if I was going to be okay. With everything I had going on medically, I couldn't risk having any emergency surgery, especially now. She said that being pregnant doesn't change anything from a Crohn's perspective. She asked that I keep her aware of how I was feeling, but also to just keep doing what I had been doing until then.

Moving into my second trimester, my OB wanted me to increase my calories by almost double what I had been used to. I told her that this would be very hard for me to do. She understood that this part was very tricky for me to do, especially being on mostly liquids and having gone through a high grade obstruction. Also, that I may have good days but other days feeling not well... and with that limited nutrition. I had given her a copy of my medical portfolio which had everything I was doing for my health... from my everyday schedule, nutrition, treatment, drugs, doctors or therapists I was seeing, to what procedures I had been through. Naturally, I had to be completely honest with her. This brought up the conversation about my treatment of using medical marijuana. As I am still dealing with the insecurity of others' judgement regarding this treatment, I couldn't help but feel a little shame because again I cared what she thought of me. To my surprise she said that they still have not found any real damaging concern with marijuana, and because it was medicinal use through a vaporizer, not smoke, that it made a huge difference. She preferred that I increase my appetite and control my symptoms by using it if that would keep me in an overall healthier state. Her concern was for me to have enough strength physically and psychologically while having the baby grow since it will take what it needs regardless. Also she wanted me to have enough strength to get me through the delivery.

I felt no judgment from her at all, and couldn't believe how much I was worried about what she was going to think of me and the treatment of using medical marijuana. She was great!

I also sought advice from a dear friend who is a pediatrician. We chatted about medical marijuana and how it could be a concern. I wanted any information and medically, I wanted to learn about any concern this could potentially bring onto a baby. She agreed with my OB as far as having my body stay in a less stressed state for myself and of course the baby. Also that if it would help increase my calorie intake, it would be fine because I would only use it when I needed to. Studies are showing that it could have an effect on a child's learning but nothing has been 100% confirmed. This is a very grey area. However if I could go without, great. That spoke volumes to me because again I cared about what she thought. This friend for the past couple years has given me some solid advice, and her opinion means a lot to me because I admire her more than words can express.

During the following appointment with my OB I told her that I hadn't smoked since Mother's Day. As much as I go through with almost everyday pain, I would try to go without and get through this pregnancy without the use of it. I didn't want to take even the smallest chance with it somehow affecting the baby. I would try harder to keep my symptoms at bay. I would become even more flawless in my nutrition and avoid almost all solids if that would help. I was ready to take as much accountability as possible. As I write this it has been over a year now since I've used medical marijuana even though it is my treatment of choice and not pharmaceutical drugs. Going through my pregnancy I had permission to do so because not only did I not abuse it, but it would help with increasing my nutritional intake, increase my energy levels, quiet my anxiety, help with sleep, aid with my symptoms, and make eating solids a little more comfortable. I couldn't help feeling that while smoking on my own was one thing, smoking while growing a baby was another. Maybe it was my own insecurity of how others would look at me using medical weed. Maybe it was a test to see if I could go without and still get through what I was dealing with. It wasn't easy and it took months to dig deep every time I thought about smoking.

While I continued with my pregnancy, I did run into painful days. I can only describe them as being a tad different from those of not being pregnant. Same cramping, contracting and stinging sharp pains. However with the extra pressure the baby was putting on my insides, it was different pain. Having the fact that I also have two areas of obstructive intestines, my situation was very different than most. As the baby grew, I felt more and more cautious of what I was eating. I could no longer feel my obstruction area as clearly as I could when I wasn't pregnant. That section of bowel felt cramping most often and I would pray that nothing would turn into an emergency surgery. I also tried to keep environmental stressors at bay, which was not easy.

From the beginning my OB had recommended that I have a caesarean. She felt that since I had perianal disease in the past, overall this would be a safer option. She preferred a vaginal birth and that there was a chance that I could do very well, however there was a higher risk for ripping that could tear my fistula, which could leave my perineum area in a horrible state should the worst happen. Also having surgery causes the immune system to react and could trigger the fistula that I already have with inflammation to become more active. There was a potential risk as well for a fistula by the incision but not likely. It was her job to make sure that not only did I understand all of the information she gave me, but also that I understood all of the negative and positive effects to both modes of delivery. As much as she was to care for the baby growing inside of me and taking the chance to have a vaginal birth, she didn't want delivery to put me into an even worse physical state. There were less complications having a caesarean and the baby would be just fine, as opposed to potentially a vaginal birth and having potentially severe complications that would leave me with more lifelong complications. As I was already living with Crohn's, adding any physical damage would be very difficult especially while caring for my baby. It was stressful to even think about having a C-section, and by no means did I want to have surgery to deliver my baby. I also didn't know that I would have to schedule the C-section a week earlier than the delivery due date. It is apparently better to not go into labour first then end up having to potentially face an emergency caesarean. I was definitely feeling pressure even though I could understand why most doctors thought it would be safer and were looking out for my health. There were no guarantees that anything wouldn't go wrong, just as much as everything vaginally would go right. I wanted to deliver vaginally, naturally, of course.

My OB, husband and I thought it best to set a date for a caesarean as I wanted to make sure my OB would be the one performing the surgery. Nothing was set in stone and it could always be cancelled down the road.

I left her office that day with a C-section scheduled for the morning of December 24, 2014. I didn't have much to say on our way home.

My husband did some research on his own and we had talked in depth about everything my OB had said. We discussed the potential outcomes with vaginal delivery versus caesarean, including why and how it could cause further complications to my health. We went over and over all of my thoughts, concerns and fears. He wanted to only support any decision that I would make and be there for me in any way that he could. He wasn't scared about my having a caesarean, and with his comfort I was able to at least think about it without having fear completely overwhelm me.

I met with my GE in late November 2014 and really needed her counsel. Even though I could very easily go through a vaginal birth and have no complications with my Crohn's, I asked if she could do an 'anal exam' and let me know, in her opinion, if my perineum area would be okay going through a vaginal birth.

After her exam she explained that I didn't just have the one non-active fistula, but that I had a smaller one as well. Though the two of them were non-active, I didn't know I had two sites. She thought it would be the safest route having a caesarean because even though I was doing great at maintaining both of them, there was no way to assure that they would not get inflamed during labour. Nor could we further investigate them because I was too pregnant to have an MRI to get a more detailed look at exactly how they looked from within the lining. Another concern was that there could be more than one tunnel which could help carry inflammation and pressure back to the original site. There was the possibility that there were many branches which would ultimately increase the risk of more inflammation and pressure. I had surgery a long time ago with one of the fistulas, but had no idea that I had a second one closer to my anus.

My GE felt that especially having not one but two non-active fistulas, I shouldn't take the risk in having them go into a worse state, which can happen even when not going through labour. Having perianal was just another health issue I was trying to manage and maintain its ongoing symptoms.

My husband and I left her office and she later sent her notes about the appointment to my OB. My head was spinning with all the information, but with my husband there to talk to, I felt comforted.

We discussed everything again, as well as this new information we just learned from my GE. I felt more comfortable thinking about having a caesarean. I felt as though I was 75% ready to make it my final decision. The other 25% was hoping I would just go into labour late enough that she would not be too early and it would be a very quick and painless vaginal delivery, one where there would be no time to make any of these hard decisions. I know I was a little in 'La La' land, but can you blame me?

The next appointment with my OB was to go over my GE's notes as well as my own. I was ready to gain as much information as I could that would help me get ready for a caesarean. I thought I would be less anxious knowing everything that the surgery and process would entail. I needed to know every little detail and I asked a lot of questions not only to my OB, but of the whole medical team that would be in the room... as well as the nurses and their responsibility. I even met with the head nurse to go over what I could expect from the nurses. From the surgery side of things I was concerned that an intern would be cutting me open and making a mistake on the incision. I was worried that they would potentially cut the baby's head. I was worried that after taking the baby out that they would not stitch me up well enough. I didn't want to be practiced on by a new intern because I already had enough going on with having obstructed pieces of bowel. I was worried that they would cut my bowel and an issue would come about with them. I had never had a catheter and didn't want to have one of those during the surgery. I was very nervous about having an epidural and something going wrong. I hated having needles and there was no way to get out of having an IV for the duration of the hospital stay. I had anxiety that I wouldn't get my baby right away. I was worried that they wouldn't remember what I wanted and go ahead, giving her the kale shot and eye drops right away when I wanted them to be delayed. I had a fear that they would take my baby away to another room and she would be crying. Having also heard traumatic stories, I was anxious about pretty much everything.

During the following appointment, my OB and the nurses that I had talked with helped put a lot of my anxiety to rest.

It was already the 2nd of December and we were weeks away from delivery. Still keeping in the back of my head that I could possibly still be lucky enough to go through a vaginal birth with zero issues, I was getting ready for a C-section, with good reason as well.

I met my OB that Tuesday like always. I had gotten my iron levels up, which she had recommend since they were low. My blood pressure and heart rate were great, as well as those of the baby's. From the ultrasound the baby was very active, which she was from the beginning. Things were looking very good, however my OB had a little concern with my pregnancy, then at 35 weeks and 5 days, since my baby was only weighing in around 4 lbs 12 oz. She wasn't overly concerned because this was the time when a baby can grow significantly, and also since ultrasounds aren't always 100% accurate regarding weight. During the last few weeks an ultrasound is preformed every week, but the weight and size of the baby is calculated every second week. She explained that the next weight for the baby would be in two weeks and hopefully she would be well over five pounds. If not, she explained that for whatever reason the baby may not be absorbing enough nutrition, and that it may be better to take the baby out a little early as she may gain more weight and do well in the outside atmosphere than inside.

I left that appointment and discussed the details with my husband. We felt assured that she would probably gain much more weight and it was nothing to worry about.

During the following appointment the next week I had another routine ultrasound and everything looked great with the baby. After that I had a monitor around my belly to check the baby's heart rate and movements. She was very active and did excellent.

My OB finished the exam and we went over the details for the following appointment, during which I would be meeting the anesthesiologist. As well, we would have the size and weight of the baby.

From this point, my husband didn't attend any of the hospital appointments. He attended them in the beginning, but with his work being really busy the hospital appointments I did on my own and was fine with that.

On December 16th, 2014, my husband didn't want me to attend this appointment alone. I'm not sure if he could feel how anxious I was to hear what her weight and size would be or if it was that if the baby was underweight he needed to be able to take in the information my OB would give us because my nerves would be shot. We arrived at the hospital by 9:00 am, which gave me just enough time to indulge in a decaf latte. We went upstairs to the ultrasound appointment at 9:15. I got on the bed like usual and then the tech put the attachment to begin the ultrasound. About ten seconds later she said she had to go and get my OB. We asked if everything was okay and she again said she had to go get my OB. A minute later my OB came into the room, looked at the ultrasound screen, and said, "Let's go, you're having the baby right now."

My husband and I were in shock and asked, "What's going on? Are you serious?" I got off the table and we followed her down the hallway and into a room. While I was being told to lie down, I had about seven medical staff around me within minutes. I had a nurse doing blood work on my left arm and the anesthesiologist putting an IV in the right one. I heard them using the term code 333, which I later learned was for having an emergency caesarean. I felt as though I was having a really bad nightmare. I had questions being thrown at me. I had paperwork being read to me that I had to sign. I had the OB who was going to perform the surgery introducing herself and the intern who would be assisting her. I was in shock, and it was mind blowing trying to talk and make sense of anything. My husband even stepped in to ask what's going on and why is she now headed into an emergency C-section. It would have been nice to know what they knew because they only speak with you after they have all consulted each other first. Very stressful.

My OB was among the crowd of people and was now in her scrubs. I asked her if she could still perform the surgery. She said she could not because she was not scheduled for the operating room that morning. However if she herself was having it done she wouldn't think twice about having anyone else do the surgery, and that fortunately I had the best team in place on that day.

I can't tell you how surreal it was to be heading into an emergency surgery and then within minutes having it cancelled. We learned that my baby's heart rate had dropped significantly, however felt blessed that once they positioned me on my side her heart rate came straight back up and we were no longer heading into an emergency surgery. We were beyond relieved, and when almost everyone who was hovered around me left I broke out in tears. My husband was by my side and reassuring me that I did so well and stayed strong. I couldn't believe what was happening and was in a state of shock.

I still had to lie in the bed and have my baby's heart rate monitored. An hour later when I had one of the head nurses come in to check on me, we were watching her face as she was looking at the monitor. She made a call to another doctor and we thought she was calling a code 333 again. She asked me to turn on my other side because the baby's heart rate had fallen again. Once I turned on my side the heart rate bounced right back up and she hung up with whomever was on the other end. I felt a huge relief because the last thing I wanted to be having was an emergency C-section.

My OB came in to talk with me and expressed her opinion to still go through with a caesarean that day because it would be very risky going home and having her heart rate drop again for whatever reason. Or worse, turn into a stillborn situation and not having medical intervention right away. My husband and I felt the same way.

Since I had breakfast only hours prior, the anesthesiologist recommended waiting until 2:30 pm for the surgery to go ahead. Given that it was no longer an emergency situation we waited. During this time we reached out to those in our lives to inform them that we were going to be having our baby girl that day. Also, my husband had to take care of his work since neither of us were prepared to have our baby that day. As there was already concern about having the baby the following week with a caesarean had her weight not gone up significantly, my OB did not see any concern in having the baby two weeks early – as opposed to one week early – especially given that her heart rate was going up and down, which could happen for different reasons. It was not a risk we wanted to take, and I was considered to be near full term at 37 weeks and five days.

I was grateful that my husband came with me to that appointment because I don't know how I would have been without him. I can still feel the anxiety inside me when I think of what I went through. I would be lying if I said it wasn't one the scariest moments in my life.

I had one of the best nurses in all my time being cared for by nurses. I kept asking her if she was going to be with me during the procedure. She was simply amazing and that really helped with my nerves. Before we knew it, it was time. They had given my husband his scrubs and then told him that they would come get him when he was allowed in the operating room. I got off the bed slowly and began my way down to the operating room. Almost at the door, the nurse saw that my husband was calling for me as he wanted to give me one more hug, reassuring that he was there and that I would be okay.

As the team introduced themselves around me I felt as though I was watching a movie. They were not talking to me, but about me to each other... which is typical procedure, I am sure, as they would introduce themselves and what their position was while in the operating room. Still I couldn't help feeling like a troubled patient instead of a woman just about to have a baby.

My epidural was administered and with amazement I handled it better than I assumed I would. As they laid me down I began to experience less feeling in my lower half. The doctor inserted the catheter and I remember asking her if she was finished because I had not felt much discomfort. Wheef! At that point I had already gone through two of the fears I had been anticipating for this procedure. Next was hooking up my intravenous. The OB then came into the room and that's when they were about to start the caesarean. I felt a little nauseous from the prophylactic antibiotics (Ancef 2 g). The anesthesiologist gave me a shot of an anti-nausea. Even though it did seem to help, I then asked her to only given me something if I asked... such as when I requested to have my pillow adjusted. They put oxygen tubes in my nose and a hair net on my head. I had a huge sterile sheet placed from under my breasts to my abdominal area just as the intern who was assisting the OB said to me, "Do you feel this? How about here?" I didn't feel anything he was doing so he said, "Okay, we are going to start the incision."

My husband was brought into the operating room and I was very relieved to finally have him by my side. He was right beside me and kept telling me that I was doing so well.

Within minutes the intern said, "Okay, we are about to meet your baby girl." The OB and assisting intern said that I should feel a lot of pressure in a minute. Waiting to feel pain or pressure, luckily I did not feel either. The OB then held up our baby so we could see her. I looked at her with a tear and thought, wow that was inside of me… she is cuter than I expected her to be.

Our baby was out and a cry was heard. She was then taken to a station right behind me and I could see her from my peripheral vision. Even though I wanted her to be put on me right away, the hospital protocol was to have the pediatrician do her exam first to see if breathing was in any way considered an issue. Within a minute of her exam our baby had delayed respiratory distress and a low heart rate. They continued positive pressure ventilation and stimulation with some drying and suctioning. She had thick white secretions. She was gurgley at birth but had good tone and an intermittent cry. Not even another minute went by and I heard them say that they were going to have to take her to the room across the hall for further treatment. My heart sank. Feeling completely helpless I told my husband to go be with her, hold her hand, and not to leave her for ANY reason.

The pediatrician came back in afterwards to tell me what was happening. She explained that my baby had most likely been experiencing TTN (transient tachypnea of the newborn) which needed a tube inserted down her throat into her tummy to help suction out liquid because she was having a hard time breathing. She needed continual positive pressure ventilation and a C-Pap machine which would give her continuous positive airway pressure. She needed an intravenous to help stabilize her glucose and needed to be kept in an incubated chamber to keep her warm.

I couldn't take in anything she was saying. All I could do was think about my little baby not being on her mother enjoying some boob and being snuggled. I never felt so numb as I did that afternoon.

They passed by with her where I was in recovery on the way to the ICU. Wheeled up beside me was this tiny little baby in an incubator with a breathing tube and an IV in her ankle. I reached my arm in to touch her little hand and felt almost emotionless. As they continued on their way my husband stayed by her side and I remained in a recovery room alone trying to feel my legs. The nurse who I absolutely loved kept putting a bottle to my breast as I had colostrum leaking about. She said it was gold and that any amount would be beneficial to my baby, especially because she wasn't yet breastfeeding. I did not want them to bottle feed her so this was good to keep. I laid there waiting to feel my legs, which I can only describe as one of the most claustrophobic feelings ever!

I felt numb yet couldn't help the tears. I kept looking at my cell phone that thank God my nurse brought to me so that my husband and I could text each other. He was worried about me and kept wanting to come see me to make sure I was okay. That's my husband, always there no matter what, supporting me no matter what, and always thinking of my well-being. I, on the other hand, told him that he had to stay with our daughter and not to leave her. I remember praying that she would be okay and that I would be there as soon as I could move my legs. Praying that she would forgive me for not being with her or giving her the birth delivery that I wanted her to have.

While I was lying there waiting for my legs to move, crying from feeling so helpless, I was able to call a good friend who just so happens to be a pediatrician. She was able to be empathetic and from her experience she could explain things in detail from a medical perspective as to why any of this had happened. It was very hard for me to take in any information, but I was grateful that she picked up her phone when she did.

A couple hours later the nurse put ice cubes on my legs and I could slightly feel the cold. Not too much later I could feel more and more. It was a huge relief that only when you go through it can you really appreciate feeling your legs. The nurse said, "Let's try getting you into a wheelchair so you can go see your baby." With the help of two nurses I managed to get into a wheelchair. On our way to the unit where my daughter was I began to feel so nauseous that I had to go back and lie down in the bed. I was escorted to my room where I felt sick from the anesthetics. I was beginning to feel depressed because all I wanted to do was hold my baby and attempt to feed her.

Hours later my dearest friend was able to come and help to relieve my husband. While I hadn't seen my baby yet, my friend was able to go and stay by her side so my husband could use the washroom. I wanted someone by her side until I could get there. We hadn't planned on having our baby that day, so my husband also needed to go home and bring our things.

Upon his arrival back at the hospital around 10:30 pm, finally I was feeling better and he wheeled me down to meet my baby girl.

I remember feeling anxious the closer we got. Then as we entered the unit where she was asleep in her incubator the nurse took her out, and with her IV attached to her little ankle still, gently put her in my arms. Right away she was looking for food, and with the help of the nurse my baby girl latched onto my right nipple and starting sucking away. My husband by our side and finally holding my daughter, I felt at peace.

She had to remain in the ICU unit for a 24-hour period to ensure that she was able to maintain her temperature and breathe on her own. She pulled through quickly and was breathing on her own before even being taken out of the ICU unit. They also had to make sure her blood sugar was regulated and would be stable. She was only due to be released the following morning.

I was advised that because she was sleeping to go and rest myself. As hard as it was to let her go I returned to my room. Not even five minutes later I got up and walked myself back to her and held her until she was cleared to go to our room the following morning.

Finally back in our private room, we all began to experience the bliss of being together.

While there were still weigh-ins to be had, hearing tests, blood sugar tests, learning to feed her, change her, learning her cries and noises, we were all together and that made everything better. Having my husband's loving support and seeing him learn to change her for the first time with our osteopath, Isabelle, was amazing. I appreciated him staying with our baby girl every minute through such a stressful time, sending me as much information as he could through text, having to go collect our things from home in a snowstorm, not sleeping and holding her so that I could try and sleep, and being so present... I will never be able to express how thankful I was to him.

I was very grateful for my best friend (R.H.) who came in to support us in every way possible. Also having such trust in her that she would meet my baby girl before I did. That she could hold her while I slept ensured I had everything that I needed. I can't express my sincerest gratitude of not only her support but her love and compassion for our daughter. A loving godmother, soulmate and a part of our family, she continually showers us with her beautiful energy, generosity and love. We will never forget how she was there for all of us during my daughter's arrival and continues to be an amazing support.

I was also blessed to have my osteopath, Isabelle, come in to the hospital to not only work on my body but also my daughter's. She came in as a loving friend. A woman of such knowledge and expertise to do this on her own free time, I felt truly blessed to have had her by my side and I will be forever grateful to her for making us such a priority.

Two days later we were finally released. I will never forget the feeling of introducing our daughter to her new home. My husband went over and above the following weeks as my recovery was slow. He took great care of us both and I will never forget how much energy he put into us. His work ethic was nothing short of amazing and he did everything possible to ensure we were okay. He was excellent with our daughter and could even change her better than me. Even though there was so much going on getting used to a new life, we had each other and I could not have been any more grateful for that.

Our daughter Blakely is now seven months old and doing splendidly. My husband was able to take paternity leave, and every day I feel blessed to have him home with us and have his support.

Even though we didn't plan on having a daughter, she has become the centre of our existence and the love of our lives.

Chapter 10

Moving Forward

Becoming someone who I admire, respect and love has been a journey. With every passing day I am more aware that being a student of self and life has been a gift. I don't know if I would ever have gone through such a transformation if I hadn't been diagnosed with Crohn's. If I hadn't been through so much pain, would I have chosen the same different and difficult path? Most people, I am sure, would not be thankful to have a diagnosis of an illness, yet for myself I am. I am thankful for what I have been able to learn and become. I am thankful for this condition because it could have been worse. I am thankful that I was able to have great help in learning to manage this condition and my situation.

In choosing to work so closely with a team of helpful professionals and choosing to be as accountable as I can, I now only speak from my own experience and not from an assumption or from what is untrue. Every day I feel blessed to be healing and taking care of my health the best that I can, and I haven't let go of my work ethic that took years to build. When my insurance company wants to know what my daily life looks like, I want to be responsible with my time and the money that I am being paid to take care of my health. I am honest with every hour, every day, and want to feel confident that I am doing everything I can for my situation. I want them to know and trust that my healing is a huge process and that I am not taking advantage of anything.

I update my daily routine/schedule on a quarterly basis and have built a medical portfolio for my own records. I give copies to my doctors and therapists to show that I am accountable, as much as I can be. Even switching to a new protein powder or a specific snack has to be documented and well-researched.

My usual daily schedule is as follows: From 4:45 to 6:30 am my first bowel movements are usually starting to process. Since having a baby this has changed a little due to the fact that I am up throughout the night, but I am hopeful that once she is sleeping more it will be more consistent. This process is critical if I want to have a decent day feeling okay, and also to be able to have some carbohydrates (solids). From 7:00 to 8:00 am this is time for meditation and exercise, which is crucial not only for my bowels, but also my physical and mental health as well. Since having my daughter my husband has been home with us for a period of time, which has been a significant help for me in trying my best to keep up with my routine. Being exhausted or unwell, not only have I been able to have his help with her, but his support and encouragement in helping me pull through hard times. Followed by breakfast, I then document my symptoms and nutrition intake. From mid-morning to mid-afternoon I usually have appointments, errands, medical exams, therapy or doctors' appointments. I also try and study nutrition from the Canadian School of Holistic Nutrition if I have the energy to do so. Of course this has all changed quite a bit since having a baby, as I have no control over how my daughter is going to feel. I am trying hard to establish a routine for her, however this is not always within my control. Most days, at this point, I am lucky to just have the energy to get through the very busy days of caring for both of us. Three years ago I also created and try to maintain a blog online which has been a great motivation. It has also helped me share my personal journey of living with Crohn's and ultimately has been a platform towards writing this book.

When I can find a little leisure time, which is now a rare occurrence, I read a variety of books... mostly psychology, self-healing, as well as different medical books about disease prevention and treatment to natural healing. I have also become obsessed about researching anything to do with health, fitness and nutrition, especially the facts behind nutrition and what my body needs to fuel itself properly. There is a lot to do in a day, and trying to keep a well-organized environment takes time and energy. This has become, of course, more difficult when having to take care of a baby full-time. I schedule a day out for myself, which has taken years to work at and achieve. Creating a lifestyle that works for me and allows me to maintain this condition while dealing with the chronic symptoms is quite a load in itself. I have learned to be very patient with not being able to be in my exact routine and allowing my daughter to be the boss. The preparation for my meals alone, which entails trying to live on an inflammatory-free diet and mostly liquids, requires more time than one would think. Taking care of my daughter full-time adds to my daily time constraints even more so. Also, especially now with a high grade obstruction and trying to keep it maintained so that it does not go into a perforation of the bowel or an emergency surgery for another obstruction.

There is so much to learn and experiment with before you can make ingredients a part of your cravings or grocery list. Being patient while living off mostly liquids and purees in order to reduce inflammation and pain requires a lot of work. By 3:00 to 4:00 pm I am physically tired, and depending on what I did that day, emotionally I can be just drained!

Physically every day is different and I don't get a day off in my full-time job. Now having two full-time jobs with caring for my daughter, I have to be very careful. I'm not complaining one bit, however, there is no break or day off where my awareness is not with how I feel or how I am going to be feeling. By choice I have decided to take this condition with such accountability that in working with my symptoms every day, it reminds me how much it takes to feel well. I have good days, yes, but nothing consistent enough that I would be able to commit to another type of work... part-time or full-time. As I am writing this paragraph, I can't help but remember how symptom-free I felt this morning as compared to now when my stomach is feeling very tight. My right lower side has a throbbing feeling and is combined with contractions. My intestines feel more cramped after eating the solids I had today, so I really have to stick with liquids and purees for the rest of the day... most likely the next couple of days as well. My stool has become looser and my rectum is throbbing from the different textures of stools, and of course, the amount of wiping.

The skin tissues are ripped around my anus, and every time I pee or sit I feel this re-ripping. Ouch! I am doing a good job with maintaining my fistulas that are non-active, however it is within these times when I pray nothing starts to flare up. One treatment that makes my perineum area, especially the anus, feel a little better is having a good soak with some Epsom salt. Then I need to make sure to put on some Vitamin E and wait out the painful times, praying nothing gets worse. When pain occurs now, in any aspect, I can't just go and take care of myself because I have my daughter to take care of, but I do the best I can until I have a free moment or two.

Though it is hard to relate with my everyday 'job' and now being a new mom on top of it, I admire and appreciate the select few who support and love me through this journey. I have a handful of people who are never afraid to ask me and put themselves out there even though my everyday life is much different than theirs. While some may assume that I am basking in my disability or still needing to try this or do that – even perhaps assuming that I want all this 'free time' – I have had to learn great patience for their ignorance. There is not one simple cure, only a puzzle that I am learning to try and put together so that I may be well. Before I learned a great deal of self-confidence, it would frustrate me why I wouldn't get the same acknowledgement or effort from others that I would give them. I have learned to simply appreciate everyone for where they stand, and accept everyone for what they do give instead of having expectations. This has been a very hard behaviour to accept, overcome and truly feel good about. I am the first to admit, I am not perfect by any means nor am I always a pleasure to deal with.

My learned behaviours, from both childhood influences and those that I have created, have in ways handicapped and enabled the ways I have chosen to look at things throughout my life. They have also influenced the choices and decisions I have made, as well as influenced the way I have chosen to react in situations or how I am with others. It hasn't been easy to accept that I have had and still have to make changes in my life. I used to get embarrassed when I would get 'pinned' for being a certain way and showing a certain behaviour, always justifying myself instead of simply listening or admitting that I may not be right or have a clue as to why I was getting so defensive. It has taken a long time but now I am able to react without feeling judged and respond by saying, "Okay, I see what you mean and I will try to work on that." This new method has worked very well and is better than how I used to get upset and take it too personally which, being insecure most of my life, was the number one reaction until now. I have learned a great deal about myself, especially through my husband who has taught me so much... and not only about myself, but the perception behind things. Since I first met him, I always found him to be someone I could learn from and listen to for hours. He was a rare find and has been my greatest friend.

I've been going through an extreme medical condition and living mostly at the mercy of a team of specialists. I've been dealing with an insurance company that every time we are in contact I feel as though I continually have to re-justify myself and my health, which has been quite the experience. This has been going on for 8 years of now, being on full-time disability and in and out of various medical appointments and procedures. I am constantly having to be evaluated and diagnosed with a few medical issues, both physically and mentally, that seem to come one after another. I must prepare for each appointment with a positive attitude no matter how nervous or upset I may feel. Knowing that I have to stay strong and be grateful that things could always be worse has definitely been a learning curve. With each appointment I gain more insight, knowledge, experience and patience not only with the doctors but with myself.

Emotionally this does, of course, get a little overwhelming at times because my medical consultations, evaluations, procedures, managing my symptoms, being patient with my anxiety and even the preparation of my nutrition as well as my daughter's, are not the only things that weigh on my mind. There are the day-to-day things of everyday life that need attention and have timelines. This includes trying to be a good wife, but also a good mother to my daughter and the care she needs. I have my own personal goals that are important for me to set time away to work on as well. I try to keep my days as simple as I can because I have more than one very important job and stress can be triggered very easily. That being said, I cannot control life. There are the tedious little things that are said or happen that are out of my control. Little disappoints or frustrations can cause stress, and I find it very challenging to always be in control of my emotions. This is a huge part of my healing. My reactions are the key to everything. For the most part they define who I am, what I have learned and where I am emotionally.

I have so much in my life to be grateful for. I have much love and support around me every day. I have close people who are compassionate, appreciative and happy to be in my life. I never thought my full-time job would be learning to be well and live every day with complications that affect my health. I didn't exactly plan on having a baby either. I look back to my previous career of wanting to become a food and beverage director in a hotel. I spent so much of my time and energy working towards different goals. I spent a lot of time over-working and taking on unwarranted stress, and worst of all not taking care of my health or my own well-being. I chose a career in which the harder you worked, the more that was expected of you instead of appreciating what you gave. Going away to college, I would not have chosen again to work in the hospitality industry. Looking back at why I made the choice to pursue the hospitality industry, it was a toss-up between three choices. Hospitality seemed like an easy in-and-out because I did not like school. I wasn't willing to try and get through something else that required better grades or a longer period of my time. I didn't have the knowledge or confidence to want anything better. I wanted to be a boss who was admired and respected by all. I desperately wanted to be acknowledged and heard. I was someone who was lucky to pass high school, but not because I was stupid. I needed more support, encouragement and acknowledgement in my life than I had received. It's unfortunate but I also know that everything has brought me to where I stand today and I am very proud of how far I have come. I am very proud of who I am.

With my husband by my side I continue happily on this journey of living through an inflammatory bowel disease and also as a new mother to our beautiful daughter.

I am worth the ongoing full-time support and feel grateful to be able to work with my health full-time. I feel blessed to have an incredible team of doctors and therapists who continually make me feel that what I do every day is in fact one of the hardest jobs there is. I feel honoured that when I am simply running a quick errand and end up having the smallest conversation with someone who is also facing struggles, that they are left feeling as though someone can empathize with them or feel heard and possibly cared for. It has become a privilege to be asked about how I do this or how I do that, especially nutritionally.

Even though there is still so much to learn medically and with my nutrition, I am eager to do so. Even though there is much to learn physically, emotionally and spiritually, I am happy embracing every moment of it. Even though I face pain more often than most, I believe that our physical body can do incredible things and healing is just one of them. Even though many believe that the disease will win in the end, and even though I don't know how I will feel in a few hours from now or tomorrow, I believe in the process. I believe in gaining incredible knowledge, being insightful and living through the experience more than I believe in the statistics.

Although I may not be like most who are getting career promotions, raises, appraisals, etc., I am present in my life. I feel joy in doing the smallest things every day. I am happier in my life now, doing what I do full-time, than I have ever been and feel incredible abundance.

Eight years ago I thought my life was over after I was diagnosed with Crohn's. Physically, emotionally and spiritually the staircase in front of me seemed impossible to climb. It brings tears to my eyes every time I stop to acknowledge and look at how far I have come through what seemed impossible to most.

Sharing my truth through this incredible journey has been one of the greatest releases of my life. As I breathe and let go, I feel peace.

I continually strive to live well while living with an inflammatory bowel disease. Every day brings about opportunities to flourish in the greatest gift of all, life itself.

Conclusion

Where I Am Now…
Years Later, Reflecting

Looking back to when I first began writing this personal journey of mine, I almost can't believe it has been four years. Eleven years ago, when I was first diagnosed with Crohn's, I definitely did not have the courage to share my truth. Nor did I have any real insight or experience to speak from. I went from sharing a few personal details through blogging, to now sharing much of what I have had to live through with this process of diagnosis. It has been an incredible awakening and for that I am truly grateful. I live my current days with gratefulness and awareness while remembering that we only have this one physical life.

From a physical standpoint, I am continuing to live with the obstruction in my small bowel. Although I have chronic inflammation, I am hoping to attain full remission with this disease. I have not had any surgery with this disease nor am I on any daily medication. I work diligently every single day with my nutrition and remain mostly on liquids and purees. I do my best with exercise and try to live every day with minimal stress. This has been more challenging since having a child, naturally.

I have become extremely disciplined with my energy and what I choose to put into my body. It has taken years, literally, to become this way of being. It is a lifestyle that has taken years to establish and be happy with.

Emotionally and spiritually I am what I am and love from a place of true emotional abundance. Thinking about how I felt in the beginning of this process, it amazes me how much things have changed. Physically, emotionally and spiritually I feel as though the ability of being able to grow has been directly related to the amount of insecurity I have been able to accept and take in my life.

One day I would like to reach a point when I can confidently say that I am in full remission.

I have come through what was a very hard transformation of self and presently stand in a space of peacefulness.

www.ingramcontent.com/pod-product-compliance
Lightning Source LLC
Chambersburg PA
CBHW031207270326
41931CB00006B/452